Health Entrepreneurship

T0143535

The potential for health professionals to learn and practice the process of entrepreneurship to improve the quality of health care and services is enormous and untapped. Health professionals witness first-hand where changes to the health system should be made and where opportunities for improvement arise, yet they are seldom associated with entrepreneurship.

Incorporating the authors' experiences leading health systems, working on the front line and supporting corporations, NGOs and accelerators that target health entrepreneurship, this book explores:

- The why, what and how of entrepreneurship – and intrapreneurship – for health professionals.
- Resources to encourage innovation by guiding the reader through an idea development process specific to the experience and working environment of health professionals.
- The areas of need, developing ideas and prototype solutions, as well as implementing, scaling and pitching entrepreneurial ideas.

An accessible and applied guide, *Health Entrepreneurship* introduces ideas about the practical delivery and implementation of entrepreneurial ideas, allowing readers to affect necessary and positive change.

Carrie R. Rich is the co-founder and CEO of The Global Good Fund, for which she was recognized as the 2016 Ernst & Young Entrepreneur of the Year. Ms. Rich previously worked in health administration. She serves on multiple boards and is an adjunct faculty member at George Washington University where she teaches Entrepreneurship for Nurse Leaders.

Mark Vernooij is a Partner at THNK School of Creative Leadership, a social enterprise that delivers executive education to build the leaders that can create the future we need and want. He serves as an expert on innovation on the World Economic Forum's Expert Network and is a regular speaker on the topics of creative leadership, entrepreneurship and innovation.

Seema S. Wadhwa is the Assistant Vice President of Sustainability and Wellness for Inova Health System. She co-founded the Lullaby Project, which has provided over 1,000 blankets to babies in the United States and around the world, and serves on the board of the US Green Building Council National Capital Region.

Contributing authors: Berend-Jan Hilberts, Mark Turrell and Menno van Dijk.

Health Entrepreneurship
A Guide

Carrie R. Rich, Mark Vernooij and
Seema S. Wadhwa

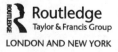

Routledge
Taylor & Francis Group

LONDON AND NEW YORK

First published 2019
by Routledge
2 Park Square, Milton Park, Abingdon, Oxon OX14 4RN

and by Routledge
52 Vanderbilt Avenue, New York, NY 10017

Routledge is an imprint of the Taylor & Francis Group, an informa business

British Library Cataloguing-in-Publication Data
A catalogue record for this book is available from the British Library

Library of Congress Cataloging-in-Publication Data
Names: Rich, Carrie R., author. | Vernooij, Mark, author. | Wadhwa, Seema
    S., author.
Title: Health entrepreneurship : a guide / Carrie Rich, Mark Vernooij, Seema
    Wadhwa.
Description: Abingdon, Oxon ; New York, NY : Routledge, 2019. | Includes
    bibliographical references and index.
Identifiers: LCCN 2018058365| ISBN 9781138564008 (hardback) | ISBN
    9781138564039 (pbk.) | ISBN 9781315122137 (e-book)
Subjects: | MESH: Delivery of Health Care—organization & administration
    | Entrepreneurship
Classification: LCC R728 | NLM W 84.1 | DDC 610.68—dc23
LC record available at https://lccn.loc.gov/2018058365

ISBN: 978-1-138-56400-8 (hbk)
ISBN: 978-1-138-56403-9 (pbk)
ISBN: 978-1-315-12213-7 (ebk)

Typeset in Sabon
by Swales & Willis Ltd, Exeter, Devon, UK

Contents

Acknowledgments

This book would not have been possible without the help of an army of supporters.

We'd like to thank our colleagues at THNK School of Creative Leadership who formed many of the theories set out in this book and who cemented them in the many articles published on www.thnk. org. Specifically, we would like to thank THNK co-founders Bas Verhart and Menno van Dijk, THNK founding dean Stefano Marzano and current dean Berend-Jan Hilberts, THNK partners Femke Bartels, Rajiv Ball and Natasha Bonnevalle, as well as the many faculty and researchers like Ton van Asseldonk, Grant Davidson, Karim Benammar, Kaz Brecher, Laurie Kemp, Lieselotte Nooijen, Mark Turrell, Robert Wolfe, Saskia Rotshuizen and Valeria Meccozi.

In our research for this book, we have met amazing health professionals and entrepreneurs who graciously shared their time to help put forward the ideas in this book. We'd like to specifically thank Floortje Scheepers, Metten Somers and Fenna Heyning.

We'd like to thank the amazing Caroline Kolar for her fearless editing and for checking our facts. Finally,

ACKNOWLEDGMENTS

none of this would have been possible without our loving parents installing in us the strength and stamina for this project: Henk and Marjolein Vernooij, Mema Lasky and Poppy Rich, Inderjit and Harpal Wadhwa. And to our loved ones who supported us while we worked through evenings and weekends: Anne Sallaerts, Darren Margolis, Nitin Sardana and the kiddos – thank-you.

Foreword

We've spent enough time in health care settings to appreciate that clinical professionals are underappreciated. We say that after having been educated as health administrators, having worked within nonprofit and for-profit health care organizations globally, and having been both caretakers and patients on multiple occasions. Clinical professionals played critical roles in each of these situations. Learning about the business dimensions of health care in both academic and professional settings forced us to think that many of the ideas the public and health professionals wrestle with could perhaps be better solved by those on the front lines of clinical care delivery.

We have had the privilege of "teaching" the content of this book to PhD nursing candidates at George Washington University. The reality is that class participants taught us more than we could possibly add to their already impressive academic knowledge base and professional experience. Through their leadership and willingness to take thoughtful risks, we tested entrepreneurship principles in the health care setting and wrestled with entrepreneurship as implemented by clinical professionals on the front lines of health care settings. We concluded that it is most important to teach and practice entrepreneurship in health care as an interdisciplinary approach, rather than approaching health entrepreneurship by practitioner type (e.g. entrepreneurship for nurses, physicians, administrators and other front-line practitioners in the health care industry). An interdisciplinary approach to entrepreneurship will enable health professionals to ultimately achieve the most successful entrepreneurial outcomes that positively impact patient care.

The health professionals who trained using the materials presented in this book developed entrepreneurial solutions to pressing problems that they faced daily in their workplaces. Their environments of practice differed, ranging from clinics to hospitals, private practices to school settings and long-term care facilities. Yet, each health professional embraced an entrepreneurial approach based on direct patient care, and shared impressive creativity when problem-solving. The health professionals in class had not previously used entrepreneurship as a vehicle for addressing health care challenges. Yet by the end of the course, every health professional had created a company or invention that he or she should be proud of. Here are examples of real testimonials from nurse leaders who participated in entrepreneurial training upon which this book is based:

Testimonials from PhD nursing candidates

"This content allowed me to think through ideas critically . . . this content was refreshing for me. I loved it."

"Thank you for taking us away from the usual nursing stuff!"

"Thanks for these pearls of wisdom and practical steps to create an idea that can change and improve health care practice. Nurses become passionate about the work and can find it challenging to translate solutions easily to those who do not work in health care . . . like investors. Getting to the point, building trust, and then creating it in a way that an investor would want to hear more and then allow for additional interactions was a key take away. My take away from the content is: this product/solution may not look the way it does today, but you can trust me to see it through to a final, useable, solution to a market need. Invaluable."

"I think this content did a lot to help us get out of our traditional habits. We could stand even more practice on how to speak to non-clinicians!"

"Time we launch this thing, I say!"

This book trains health professionals in well-established processes that empower health professionals to identify areas of need, develop ideas, prototype solutions, pitch ideas and eventually implement and scale entrepreneurial solutions. This book empowers health professionals to develop their entrepreneurial ideas, enact positive change within their work environments and demonstrate value day-to-day. While there is a clear need for innovation and change at the level of the health care systems, this book is designed to help staff in the front line to create innovation and change in their immediate context.

Health professionals who embrace entrepreneurship will directly benefit patients, colleagues and the organizations they serve. Clinical professionals have unique perspective within health care because of their on-the-ground experience directly engaging with patients, caregivers, physicians, hospital staff and third parties. This direct experience with varied customer groups enables clinical professionals to clearly identify issues and potential opportunities previously unknown to or ignored by other members of the health care system. Clinical professionals who use the entrepreneurial learnings gleaned from this book will have the tools to affect change real-time through entrepreneurial thinking.

Health professionals could be highly entrepreneurial within their workplaces, but often lack the tools and platform required to realize their ideas. Further, clinical standards that require careful adherence to checklists validated by third parties are necessary dimensions of excellent health care practice, yet reinforce the opposite approach of entrepreneurial thinking, which is founded on implementing creative approaches to problem-solving. This book provides health care professionals with the tools, knowledge and practice to develop and implement entrepreneurship in the workplace.

This book tailors entrepreneurship training to the health profession through case studies designed to address specific needs as each reader navigates the creation of his or her own product, service or company.

The case studies woven throughout this book explore entrepreneurship through the lens of health professionals by offering practical, creative approaches to entrepreneurial thinking in the health setting. Health professionals who read this book will experience entrepreneurial thinking that ranges from the initial step of identifying a health care issue or opportunity to creating a proposed product, solution, new process and even a new company. Health professionals who implement the practices gleaned from this book will positively impact their workplaces through entrepreneurship – a differentiator for clinical professionals. This book builds on methodologies and best practices from diverse industries and explains why such thinking is relevant within the health landscape.

In writing this book, we are greatly indebted to those that went before us: our teachers, mentors, the great thinkers that developed many of the processes mentioned in this book. In many ways, this book is an augmented collection of articles that were written by colleagues at THNK School of Creative Leadership, in particular THNK Dean Berend-Jan Hilberts, THNK research fellow Mark Turrell and THNK co-founder Menno van Dijk. These articles can all be found on www.thnk.org.

Chapter 1

Introduction to entrepreneurship

How does business training differ from entrepreneurship training differ from clinical training? Business training focuses on management excellence. Entrepreneurship training focuses on product, service and business design. Clinical training focuses on practice, experience, replication and memorization. In direct contrast, the training of health personnel does not reward innovation or entrepreneurship – just the opposite, in fact, it rewards accreditation and checklists.

Unlike a business book that's focused on management, this book focuses on entrepreneurship. Unlike a design book that focuses on product design, this book focuses on business design. Consider this book a resource to explore topics such as innovation practices, business design thinking, leadership development, entrepreneurial mind-set, systems thinking and societal impact. The processes in this book integrate elements used by architects, engineers, entrepreneurs, designers, strategy consultants and systems designers and business developers. This make this book's approach to entrepreneurship for health care interdisciplinary by design.

We're not just talking entrepreneurs in startups. We see entrepreneurship as a mind-set, process and a set of practices that health care personnel in the frontline – think doctors, clinicians, nurses and support staff – can use to generate solutions and innovations in their daily work.

That context is why this book spends significant time on not just the tools and practices of entrepreneurship, but also what it requires from you as a leader: the entrepreneurial mind-set. This mind-set is ultimately what will accelerate your entrepreneurial project within a health workplace. Through the topics discussed on the pages that follow, you will strengthen competencies to generate new ideas and turn them into a viable new product, service or entrepreneurial solution within your existing health care workplace.

* * * * *

We know, you're not used to thinking of yourself as an entrepreneur.

Clinical professionals are not conventionally perceived as entrepreneurs, nor do they typically think of themselves as entrepreneurs. Yet clinical professionals are perhaps the most undervalued, best kept entrepreneurial secret within the health care industry! Clinical personnel are front and center when it comes to providing clinical care, iterating what does not work and interacting with customers: patients, caregivers, physicians and other clinicians. Clinical professionals have an intimate understanding of the ecosystem in which they operate as well as the specific actors who contribute to patient health. Yet, the entrepreneurial ideas of clinical professionals are often underdeveloped, ignored, disposed by the wayside or taken by others.

The health care environment is not always conducive to entrepreneurship. The constant pressure of the next patient, the omnipresent sound of the pager, the weight of important decisions and the ever-mounting volume of work do not always allow for the more contemplative states needed for new ideas and innovation to come about. Also, essential health care concepts like safety first, protocols, directives and evidence-based care can rob us from the opportunity to prototype, experiment and learn. Finally, the increasing costs of the system, constant understaffing and overregulation remove the freedom to move, to try new things, to tinker and be entrepreneurial.

This book presents an opportunity to challenge habits and explore the edges of possibility that surround the health workforce through a proven and structured process called the Innovation Flow. This is a process that can be used to recontextualize problems in the health system and problem solve using entrepreneurship. It is a platform for improving health care in a different way from what we know to date and on a different scale than that to which health professionals are traditionally accustomed to.

This book presents a process to innovate with an accompanying tool kit to tackle complex health care challenges and create breakthrough solutions. The focus of this book is not the supply of financial capital, although an adequate supply of funds is important for health entrepreneurship long term; the focus of this book is training health professionals to think entrepreneurially. Readers are encouraged to harness and deploy entrepreneurial ideas and practical entrepreneurial solutions to pressing health care problems. You will be challenged to explore the framework and apply it to case studies as well as in your daily work. The resulting entrepreneurial approaches are reader-generated, deployable solutions to make patient care and the health care ecosystem more effective.

This book unites the concepts of health care, entrepreneurship, design thinking, strategic thinking and systems thinking. At a base level, this book gets health professionals on board with entrepreneurship and spreads entrepreneurial concepts that will work for, rather than against, clinical providers. Upon completion of this book, readers will not just know how to create and organize entrepreneurial opportunities, they will have come up with new entrepreneurial opportunities that are relevant in their context.

This book is one step toward closing the gap between health care challenges and the abundantly untapped resource of health entrepreneurship. Imagine how health care will be when professionals working within the industry live their full potential as entrepreneurs!

Chapter 2

Innovation Flow

We'll explore the topic of entrepreneurship in health care through the Innovation Flow. The Innovation Flow consists of four phases: Sensing, Visioning, Prototyping and Scaling. The Innovation Flow is the structured process that can help you develop your entrepreneurial ideas for the health industry. This chapter kick-starts your entrepreneurial journey as you:

- learn about the Innovation Flow and its four phases;
- get introduced to the different;
- leverage your learning into a Creative Question.

At the end of this chapter, you will understand what the Innovation Flow is, what its elements are and how to use it. We will conclude this chapter by letting you define a problem or challenge that you would like to solve using health entrepreneurship.

Introduction to the Innovation Flow

The hallmark of the creative artist is to create something that did not exist before, perhaps a painting, a sculpture or an idea. This generative capacity is not limited to artists: entrepreneurs and corporations conceive and create new products, services and platforms that did not previously exist. Our complex, accelerating and volatile world needs this creative ability now more than ever, especially in all levels of health organizations.

So how well do we understand this ability to create and implement new ideas? What competencies are required to do so? Is the best training ground for entrepreneurship in business or design school or some other vehicle for learning? Maybe it is a school where creativity and leadership blend. Understanding creative leadership means understanding creativity. Few of us create alone today. As Keith Sawyer shows in *Group Genius*, there is a persistent myth of the lone inventor, one great genius tinkering in obscurity (Sawyer, 2017). But this is, indeed, a myth.

Innovation usually comes from group interaction, from cross-fertilization between team members and from rapid feedback cycles. Creativity happens in teams. As Pixar Animation Studios' President Ed Catmull points out, the team is even more important than the idea. A great team will either turn a mediocre idea into a great movie or jettison it, but a mediocre team will waste a great idea (Catmull, 2008). A great team can start with an average idea and be creative on the way, changing it as they go along.

Innovation and creativity are important. Entrepreneurship is imperative. Entrepreneurship is often, though not always, founded on innovation and creativity. Think of entrepreneurship as the vehicle to implement ideas, often in innovative and creative ways that meet market demand.

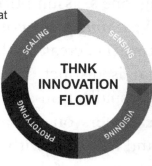

Design into the concept a few small smart moves that will increase the odds for the concept to have an outsized impact

Conduct a wide exploration of the topic, combining rational analysis with intuitive and associative gathering of insights

Perform iterative and rapid user testing and feedback loops to improve the concept

Create breakthrough concepts by thinking big, reframing beliefs and using analogies

FIGURE 2.1 THNK Innovation Flow

Innovation combines the concept for a new product, service or business and the team behind it, led by a powerful leader. These major elements begin by the genesis of an innovative concept and describing it. Realization consists in giving birth to this idea in the form of an enterprise.

The enterprise concept is developed in a cycle which consists of Sensing, Visioning, Prototyping and Scaling, otherwise known as the Innovation Flow (THNK School of Creative Leadership, www.thnk. org). This flow is designed as a cycle because of its iterative nature: often entrepreneurs have to go back to where they started to solve problems they didn't know existed or to capture an opportunity in a slightly different way than when they started out.

The first phase – called *Sensing* – consists of a wide exploration of the topic, combining rational analysis with an intuitive and associative process of gathering insights. This process includes observing the user (an external user like the patient or their relative or an internal user like a doctor or nurse) in his or her habitat, rethinking one's assumptions and engaging with the user. The *Visioning* phase consists of reframing the issue and ideating (i.e. creating through iterations) a new concept that is distinct, bold and appealing, through synthesis, visualization and articulation. The *Prototyping* phase centers on repeated experimentation, user testing and feedback with the aim of testing one's assumptions to improve the concept.

Scaling, the final phase, is about designing for scalability. Scalability means different things in different contexts. Scalability at the individual level is the ability to have impact beyond one's own reach. At the organizational level, scalability is an idea that spreads quickly and gets adopted by many. At the enterprise level, it is a concept that can be multiplied at little or no additional cost. That last point is important. We all know that health systems need to control spending, so the ability to employ entrepreneurial solutions that save money or generate new income for the health care organization is important for entrepreneurial ideas to gain traction.

Entrepreneurs aim for their concepts to be designed for maximum potential scale and impact. Many times, though not always, scalable concepts are digital or online to leverage technology. As we further explore entrepreneurship, one might consider what unique challenges digital solutions present within the health care industry.

Scalable concepts can be based on do-it-yourself tools; for example, selling recipes is more scalable than running a restaurant. Scalable concepts are based on virality and advocacy instead of advertising.

Scalability translates directly into business performance. The most precious case of a scalable concept is one that feeds on itself over time. A commerce platform – stock exchange, online marketplace, buying cooperation – offers ever better deals as it attracts more volume and members.

Do not be put off by these entrepreneurial ideas from the food, finance or online industries if they seem out of line with your health care experience. Health entrepreneurship will benefit from exposure to entrepreneurial thinking that is interdisciplinary, thinking that has worked well in other industries and can be applied in the ripe-for-disruption health care industry.

The Innovation Flow in health care

The health care industry faces challenges that at times feel insurmountable because of their complexity. The Innovation Flow is an approach to tackling those challenges that are difficult to solve. Traditional, deductive, linear problem-solving approaches typically fail in such settings or result in solutions that address only part of the problem.

Health care challenges often come with high degrees of uncertainty and low degrees of predictability for a variety of factors, such as dependency on technology development, the environment and socioeconomics. Challenges in health care consist of interconnected and interdependent sub-issues. These issues must be tackled collectively and, frequently, simultaneously. Health challenges involve multiple stakeholders who affect one another and health in sometimes unpredictable ways.

Trial and error will be part of your entrepreneurial process – a difficult reality to swallow when human life is involved. We'll learn more about how to safely and effectively navigate this process as we dive deeper into the Innovation Flow.

As health professionals, you know well the importance of investigating a problem in its full context with inclusion of all stakeholders involved, but first and foremost the immediate users – patients. With that background, we must accept that entrepreneurship is explorative and provides no guarantee that a solution will be found. Many times, the entrepreneurial process leads to surprise findings that invariably disappoint stakeholders who may have a preferred solution already in mind. Further, the team members involved in the entrepreneurial process have a significant influence on the outcome of the process. The entrepreneurial process will likely produce unique outcomes based on the composition of the team that conceived the outcomes. As in most every other setting, choose your team members carefully!

Simple solutions may or may not be within reach to address health care problems. The Innovation Flow is an entrepreneurial process that is especially useful where standard solutions (which may or may not be simple) previously failed. Challenges in health care are often so complex that it's difficult to define where such problems start or end. We will explore processes in this book to reframe challenges that alter or broaden ways of thinking about the problem at hand, which creates space for finding novel and creative solutions. The most effective way to familiarize oneself with entrepreneurial tools and methodology is to explore entrepreneurship in a sequential manner, keeping in mind that very little about entrepreneurship in practice is linear, sequential or rigid.

Entrepreneurship in action: a superhero Superformula

The A.C. Camargo Cancer Center had an insight that intravenous bags are perhaps one of the more depressing sights around. Another insight was that getting kids hooked up to them was very stressful to the children and their family and, as a result, time-consuming. Finally, the first step in the fight against a disease is believing in the cure. But the chemotherapy is extremely difficult, especially for a child.

The team, consisting of hospital staff, people from creative agency JWT and Warner Bros., explored whether they could solve the user need of making the chemotherapy process easier and providing children extra strength while undergoing treatment. They realized that superheroes are typically the essence of strength and this fueled their Creative Question: how might we transform chemotherapy into a "Superformula"?

They developed the concept of Superformula: a new chemotherapy experience, aimed at raising kids' spirits and make them feel stronger. They created simple plastic covers with logos from the *Justice League* characters like Batman and Wonder Woman that go over the intravenous bags.

(continued)

(continued)

Prototyping with hospital staff led them to create covers that are easy to sterilize and meet hospital standards. In conjunction, they created a comic book series where kids can see and read about these same superheroes as they battle cancer and recover successfully and bravely. Finally, the entire children's ward was redesigned to fit the theme, with superheroes, a Hall of Justice and an exclusive entrance that fits a hero's welcome.

Challenge: topic, team and environment

We are going to break the Innovation Flow apart to explore what the process looks like and how to navigate it for a health professional approaching entrepreneurship for the first time. Entrepreneurship is not solely about knowledge; it consists of knowledge of the process, skills to apply the process with concrete tools and the relevant mind-sets. This means that it's also about practicing these skills and training these mindsets. It's about doing rather than just thinking. For the sake of making entrepreneurship accessible, we want you to apply the learning from this book to a concrete case. So, let's start with what we know. Identify an issue at work that frustrates you. What in your work ticks you off? What problem or opportunity keeps you up at night? What infuriates you? Or what solution have you always wanted to bring to the world?

This is what we call the challenge: the case, issue or opportunity that you use to practice the innovation phases on for the duration of this book, so choose a challenge you care about deeply. We will revisit this challenge at the end of each chapter.

While entrepreneurship can feel like a lonely and uphill battle, it's not something to do alone. To understand the full context of your challenge through Sensing, you will need diverse perspectives. To come up with ideas you need to co-create them with others. To prototype your ideas and scale them, it's helpful to work together with others and get their support. This means you need a team. Knowing which individuals will make creative sparks fly together is a mix of art and science that often comes from a gut instinct.

Three key elements to consider when building your entrepreneurial team are:

CREATIVE TEAM BUILDING CHECKLIST

Knowing which individuals will make creative sparks fly together is a mix of art and science, that often comes from a gut instinct.

SIMILAR CALIBER

For the team to challenge each other, the team members need to be well matched. They need to be able to look each other in the eye, disagree where they see fit, and challenge one another on issues rather than emotions or personalities. The creative leader can be a member of the team he or she casts. In this case, it is even more critical to be surrounded by equally strong-willed team members, in order to avoid the de facto creation of an operational team.

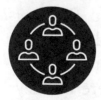

CO-CREATION ABILITY

The team members need to have a sufficiently compatible approach to the creative process, including the ability to listen to and build on each other's ideas, to embrace mistakes as opportunities, to let go of what is not working and to not be 'married 'to ideas or take criticism vpersonally. This includes a sufficient level of commonality in culture and work ethic to quickly establish trust and one working language. But be careful not to create a team of "Yes Men" either.

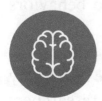

DIVERSITY OF THOUGHT

At the heart if the creative team-building process is combining hitherto unrelated ideas brought to the table by people from a wide array of backgrounds. It is absolutely vital that creative leaders bring together teams that represent differences in outlooks, expertise levels, and ways of thinking. Without the right mix people, the entire effort becomes one man's burden. In essence, the team members need to be able to surprise each other to produce the best results.

FIGURE 2.2 Elements of successful entrepreneurial teams

We need to be clear here: we are speaking about creative teams, not operational teams. An operational team looks to solve defined problems with known solutions. A creative team works on understanding and rearticulating the problem itself first and then searching for solutions that are unknown or unconventional. When a creative team has come up with a solution and has fully developed a concept, it can hand over the solution to an operational team for execution, or the creative team itself can become the operational team.

The optimal size for a creative team is three. Anything smaller lacks the diversity to generate creative perspectives, and will seem under-resourced. Larger teams suffer from complexity of coordination. Experience teaches us that when a four-five person team struggles to make progress and complains about the workload, it works best to reduce its size, not reduce the scope or postpone the deadline, and certainly not to add even more team members.

Five years ago, Google became focused on building the perfect team (Rozovsky, 2015). In Silicon Valley, software engineers are encouraged to work together, in part because studies show that groups tend to innovate faster, see mistakes quicker and find better solutions. After looking at over a hundred groups for more than a year, Google concluded that understanding and influencing group norms were the keys to improving teamwork. They noticed two behaviors that all the good teams generally shared:

- First, **on the good teams, members spoke in roughly the same proportion,** a phenomenon the researchers referred to as "equality in distribution of conversational turn-taking." Some teams saw everyone speaking during each task, while others saw a shift of leadership among teammates from assignment to assignment. But in each case, by the end of the day, everyone had spoken roughly the same amount. "As long as everyone got a chance to talk, the team did well," Woolley said. "But if only one person or a small group spoke all the time, the collective intelligence declined" (www.cs.cmu.edu/~ab/Salon/research/Woolley_et_al_Science_2010-2.pdf).

- Second, **the good teams all had high "average social sensitivity"** – a fancy way of saying they were skilled at intuiting how others felt based on their tone of voice, their expressions and other nonverbal cues. One of the easiest ways to gauge social sensitivity is to show someone photos of people's eyes and ask him or her to describe what the people are thinking or feeling – an exam known as the "Reading the Mind in the Eyes" test. People on the more successful teams scored above average on the Reading the Mind in the Eyes test. They seemed to know when someone was feeling upset or left out. People on the ineffective teams, in contrast, scored below average. They seemed, as a group, to have less sensitivity toward their colleagues.

Other behaviors were deemed important as well – making sure teams had clear goals and creating a culture of dependability. But Google's data indicated that, above all, psychological safety was critical to making a team work.

15

So before you start Sensing, think about which two people in your environment would be good to team up with and see if you can get them to join your journey.

Finally, entrepreneurship requires the right environment. You want to create space and time that allow for reflection, exploration and co-creation. This means you have to find an environment where there is not the constant interruption of the pager and daily disturbances. Preferably an environment where you can create a canvas or visual overview with everything you learn (think Post-it's research finding, pictures, flip charts). Talking about Post-its, we urge you to use sticky notes (from any brand) to capture things you learn on the way. The advantage is that you can reorganize and cluster them all the time. To create Post-its that are eligible for others and that still make sense even after not having seen them for a while, there are some golden rules to writing a good Post-it versus a bad Post-it.

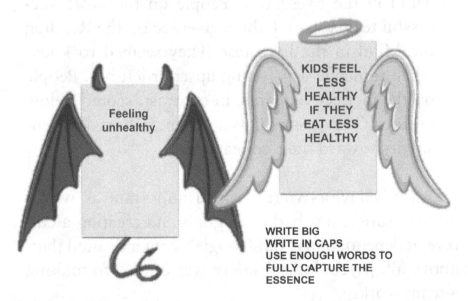

FIGURE 2.3 Post-it best practices

Chapter 3

Sensing

Explore the problem

This chapter provides a more in-depth look at the first phase of the Innovation Flow, Sensing (van Dijk & Hilberts, 2014). The Sensing phase of the Innovation Flow focuses on understanding entrepreneurship with an open mind and a willingness to explore problems and opportunities in the context of health care from as many perspectives as possible. This chapter guides your entrepreneurial journey as you:

- discover insights;
- cultivate a deeper understanding of users;
- identify interactions, movement and unarticulated needs;
- expose conventional wisdom to find entrepreneurial insights;
- leverage your learning into a Creative Question.

At the end of the Sensing chapter, you will understand the concept of Sensing, you will have explored the required mind-sets and you will have worked on a challenge of your choosing with tools from the Sensing tool kit (Hilberts, 2018). We will conclude this chapter by transforming the challenge you identified in Chapter 2 (remember: that problem, opportunity or issue that keeps you up or bothers you) into a Creative Question that begs for a creative and entrepreneurial solution.

Introduction to Sensing

The Sensing phase of the Innovation Flow is the first phase to understanding the challenge you'd like to address in health care. The Sensing phase is when team members conduct a wide exploration of the topic. Rational analysis is combined with an intuitive and associative process of gathering insights. Sensing starts with curiosity. We face something familiar with a fresh perspective that enables us to gain new insights into old problems.

The essentials for the Sensing phase are exploring the unknown, looking for perspectives that don't look like they often go together and identifying the unarticulated user needs. Challenge conventional wisdom. You're looking for original insights during the Sensing phase. Keep in mind that you don't know what you're looking for until you've found it, so be patient.

The art of Sensing entails taking a few steps back before solving an innovation question to identify fresh insights that can spark breakthrough ideas later. All too often, we dive into solving a problem or brainstorming a solution without true understanding of the complexity of the problem, the true needs of those involved and without first finding some new insights into the problem at hand. Sensing requires exploratory thinking to get a broad and different perspective on the initial problem or situation. Sensing is not efficient. It is not a straight path of finding what you need. Instead it is an often-frustrating search along several paths. You are making the journey to discover what you do not know yet. This makes it hard: you are looking for something you do not know. Therefore, its success greatly depends on the diligence and discipline of the expedition. The right mind-set is that of an explorer who sets foot on new land for the first time.

During Sensing, you want to collect unexpected treasures and insights that will help you look at the problem from a new, original angle. To be specific, you're looking for insights and user needs. Insights are objective facts about the situation. They can be in the form of statistics or surprising things you didn't know. The more surprising the insight, the less people know it, the more interesting it is. User needs on the other hand are more subjective, they are personal to a specific individual or group of individuals. User needs can be articulated, i.e. clearly stated by a user (e.g. "I want a cheap vegetable isle in the supermarket") or unarticulated (e.g. "I want to have access to cheap vegetables in order to eat healthy"). They can also be factual (e.g. "I want to eat healthy to stay fit") or emotional (e.g. "I want to eat healthy to feel better around my friends"). The more emotional the user need is and the more unarticulated, the more interesting it typically becomes. Better and different ideas will eventually be the result but they are not the goal of Sensing.

Entrepreneurship in action: Sensing the problem of infant mortality

High death rates among premature born babies are a big problem in India. Initially, it was presumed that baby incubators were too expensive for families and hospitals to afford, so hospitals and product developers worked together to design lower-cost incubators targeted for developing markets. Yet after conducting more thorough research on user experience by immersing themselves with the families, they realized that the problem wasn't that simple. Costs were not the problem – access to hospitals was. Indian mothers living in rural areas delivered at home and could not reach hospitals in time.

Indian mothers were asking for baby incubators but instead were helped by low-cost infant sleeping bags that helped keep their premature babies alive. Embrace Warmer (www.embraceinnovations. com) is a simple, portable infant sleeping bag heated with a wax-like substance that remains at body temperature for hours. This well-known success case is often attributed to "customer intimacy": being close to the user. But notice, when asked, mothers and doctors could not have stated their user need as at-home incubators in the form of infant warmers did not yet exist. The unstated need "keep my baby warm" was way more important than the stated need "have access to a low-cost incubator."

Note that while you're Sensing, your brain will inevitably come up with ideas and solutions. We're not looking for these right now as we're only looking for insights and user needs. So, write your ideas down and park them. You might need them later and by parking them, you free your brain from carrying them around and create room for more observations.

This pursuit of Sensing is a disciplined process. It takes discipline to:

- commit enough time and resources;
- apply different lenses if you want to find new treasures;
- postpone judgment and stay away from forming initial ideas if you want to learn something new;
- capture the treasures you collect on the way.

Sensing leverages the powers of intuition and analysis, and unlimited curiosity, and puts a bonus on the capability to challenge conventional wisdom and rethink the world around us.

Pointers to embrace while you're Sensing: stay curious and naïve by looking at scenarios through new eyes. At the same time, think critically, analytically and intuitively. Try to empathize with your users and be patient (no pun intended). Recognize serendipity so that you are open to and accept ambiguity from your findings.

What should be the outputs at the end of the Sensing phase? The outcome will not look like your typical medical notes; you should have a scrapbook with dozens of varied insights and user needs. You might choose to capture these insights on the wall, they could take the form of images you print, magazine clippings, research data, patient or colleague testimonials, sketches, etc. The goal is to physically see your Sensing phase. The outcome of your Sensing phase should be a diverse array of inspiration and insights – a handful of original insights, compelling user needs and original perspective on the challenge, pointing toward a solution.

When eventually you look over all those insights and start Connecting the Dots, new patterns will emerge that point toward a clearer question or a solution direction. Sensing ends with synthesizing to discover amongst all collected material the most original insights and most compelling user needs. It then converges upon a restatement of the initial problem in the form of a Creative Question. A well-formulated question that begs to be answered and points toward a solution space that is pregnant with potential. This Creative Question is the springboard into the Visioning phase.

Sensing is disciplined

Where do you start when you want to improve the health system? Do you start jotting down ideas? Do you grab a whiteboard and Post-its, get a few people in the room and start brainstorming? Whether the aim is an incremental change or a disruptive solution, don't jump to solve the problem right away.

Health entrepreneurship means approaching the topic from a new perspective. Health professionals need to set aside their well-practiced skill of pattern recognition. Take a few steps back and do a rigorous exploration of the problem, as if you are an explorer and setting foot on new land for the first time.

When launching on a quest for breakthrough ideas, entrepreneurship feels quite like exploring uncharted territory. Like an explorer in new territory, you may have a sense of direction and an overall goal, yet you are making the journey to discover what you do not know yet. This makes it hard: you are looking for something you do not know. Therefore, its success greatly depends on the diligence and discipline of the expedition.

The word discipline is not used lightly here. We have learned from guiding health entrepreneurs in their Sensing activities that it takes discipline to:

- commit enough time and resources to see the situations you have seen before in a totally new way and to explore new situations;
- apply different lenses if you want to find new treasures;
- postpone judgment and stay away from forming initial ideas if you want to learn something new;
- capture the treasures you collect on the way diligently.

How much time and resources do we devote before we start to come up with answers? It is tempting to jump right in when given a problem. You think you see the answer already. Health entrepreneurship means understanding that it's not that the first answers are bad, it's that they are *incremental*. They build on what you already know about the topic and this takes time and resources. Of course, there are competing commitments so it might feel counterintuitive to carve out time for Sensing in your calendar. Clinicians rarely do this for themselves, which is where health entrepreneurs come in, through forcing teams to do Sensing and allocating enough resources to do so. It takes time to win the trust of the users you are observing and interviewing, to study the facts and the figures and to sift through material and dig up the few nuggets of gold.

Look through different lenses

When Sensing, you are looking to develop a fresh perspective and identify weak signals. Health entrepreneurship entails discovering as many different insights as possible. This process requires using different lenses. The microscope to zoom in on the details, get an up-close-and-personal view of your user: what does she do, say, think and feel? The telescope to zoom out on the full context of the problem, who else is involved, what are the Force Fields in the ecosystem, what has been done in the past, what are the facts?

Throughout this book, we will use the problem of encouraging people to eat more fruit and vegetables as an example. When working at this problem in the Sensing phase, one could explore dining habits, such

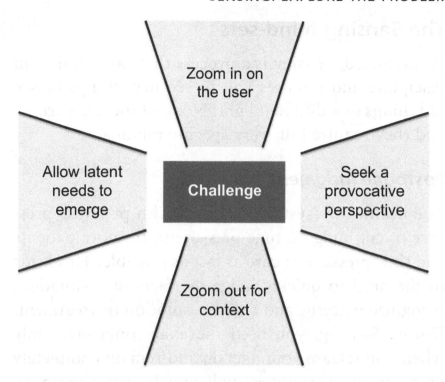

FIGURE 3.1 Sensing takes multiple lenses

as the disappearing ritual of the family discussion over dinner. Or explore different cooking styles and recipes. One can delve into different consumer segments, different types of potential restaurant visitors and different unmet needs. One can explore different brand images on food packaging. One can look at the topic from a business angle, looking at the profitability of different formats. One can take an engineer's perspective looking for new ways to get to maximum throughput in the produce production industry. One can take the perspective of a real estate planner, looking for new concepts that various farmers' market locations might trigger. Or one can take a technology angle using new techniques to prepare food or select food ingredients that are produced in "advanced" ways.

The Sensing mind-sets

As discussed, Sensing is a process that takes time and discipline and requires you to see new things or see old things in a different light. None of these are trivial and they require four very specific mind-sets:

Postpone judgment

The health care system is riddled with pressure: pressure to cut budgets, time pressure to fit more patients and time pressure to cure as fast as possible. This leads to the need to quickly judge the facts of a situation, recognize patterns and define a solution or treatment. During Sensing, you need the exact opposite. Only when you release your agenda and remain completely open to all possibilities, will you be truly receptive to new learning. This is exceptionally hard to do for people who work in result-oriented, time-pressured environments – i.e. health care. Yet health entrepreneurship means knowing that the moment you believe you know the answer or form a judgment, you will be obstructing the view of the unexpected, and risk missing out on serendipitous encounters.

Truly listening without judging is not an easy task. It helps to force yourself to listen for what you do not want to hear. For instance, if a team is excited about a new opportunity space, it might be tempted to close its ears to those saying, "we tried that already in the past and it failed." However, if you force yourself to listen, you have an interesting Sensing opportunity to delve into experience and draw learning from it. The other way around, the fact that you didn't succeed in solving a certain situation before does not mean you can't find a different way to solve it today.

Cherish the not knowing

Health professionals are often consulted for their knowledge and experience. Their knowledge is often the basis of the trust that patients have. This puts huge pressure on health professionals to know the answer or at least to not come across as if they don't know the answer. For health entrepreneurship, to find what you are *not* looking for, you must start by asking truly open questions, and questions that might feel like dumb questions or questions you already think you know the answer to. Overcoming this discomfort and even cherishing it is key to truly seeing the new. Empathy is at the core of the Sensing phase. When the questions are asked in a caring way, they will help win you the trust of the interviewee and possibly reveal pain points that can lead to crucial insights.

Challenge the confirmation bias

Instinctively human beings want to be right. Most health professionals are good at learning and being right. They had to study very hard to get where they are and continue to study to stay there. For these top students it's even more of a reflex to want to be right. Unfortunately, this creates a tendency to focus on the data, information or stories that confirm our hypothesis instead of looking in detail into the reasons why we might be wrong in our hypothesis. For example, when looking at data we typically disregard the "outliers" and only look at the trends. In entrepreneurship, however, the most interesting stories and the best insights might be in these outliers. That's where opportunity is hiding.

Patience, patience, patience

It's very rewarding to generate solutions to a problem. Our entire education system – in which many health care professionals have spent significant time – is geared toward only rewarding solutions. Sensing, however, does not bring you any solutions; if done well, it just brings more questions. Committing to Sensing before starting to generate ideas is therefore counterintuitive for many, especially for natural "converters" who want to get to the answer right away. However, when the aim is improving health care, health professionals know that it requires time and significant patience to "diverge" and explore.

Entrepreneurship in action: the Aravind Eye Hospitals and Clinics

India, unfortunately, is known for being the country that has the largest blind population in the world. Many of those that that are blind are dealing with cataracts, which is a treatable simple surgery. Unfortunately much of the population cannot afford this treatment. Cataracts are the leading cause of blindness in India, although glaucoma and diabetes-related blindness are also treatable and expensive. Two-thirds of the blind population are within Asia and, of those two-thirds, three-quarters reside in India. Access to affordable health care is critically necessary however, and not always achieved. Additionally, access to affordable health care should not come at a compromise to the quality of that care.

The Aravind Eye Hospitals and Clinics are a health care chain in India founded by Dr. Venkataswamy (Dr. V) in 1976. Although it started as a single location. That single location was started by Dr. V mortgaging his entire life savings. It had 11 beds, with six that were reserved for paying patients and five that were for nonpaying patients (Rosenberg, 2013). Over the years it has grown into a network of hospitals and clinics across India focused on eradicating cataract-related blindness. By 2012, Aravind had treated nearly 32 million patients and performed four million surgeries. It has been a driving force in supporting the blind in India. The Aravind Eye Hospitals and Clinics in India revolutionized the entire system of providing eye surgeries, with astonishing results both in financial terms and in terms of health outcomes. Solving for this large scale solution called for thinking about the problem from a different perspective.

What makes the Aravind model very unique was their roots of Sensing during the very early phases. The foundation rested on looking at care delivery models through the heart and emotionally connecting to those the clinic was aiming to serve. That needed to be tied, of course, to a business model but clear in the Sensing was the insight that many could not afford the care they so desperately needed. Also, many were suffering from blindness that was completely treatable. The founder of the clinic was very connected to the patients he aimed to serve.

One of the keys to success for the clinic includes not only engaging with the community but truly partnering with them. This includes creating eye-care community camps. These camps are organized by the community themselves. They support the logistics of finding a location as well as volunteers. Critical resources from the clinic are focused on doing their part – checking division rather than focusing on the logistics of the event. Each part of the care is isolated from the pre-check, to the doctor's analysis, to the eye testing and checking for glaucoma. The doctor ultimately takes all of the information and makes a final analysis and prescribed treatment. Glasses are provided right there on the camp site. Individuals get to choose the frames of their choice. This is critically important, as they learned in Sensing, to drive adherence to actually using the glasses. For those who require surgery, there are buses waiting and taking individuals on the spot to the base hospital. The logistical support is critical to a smooth operation but also for the end user as it significantly increases their likelihood of taking action. Surgeries are provided the following day. Patients are discharged within a few days and returned back to their home communities where they will be cared for. There are several thousand camps each year.

The roots of success stemmed from a desire to model eye-care delivery in the same ways as McDonald's offers food. Looking at delivering eye surgeries in the same way hamburgers are delivered really was a breakthrough idea. It was uncharted territory and lead to making a discovery on how to do things differently. We will learn more about this strategy in our chapter on Visioning.

Unfortunately, even with all of the success the clinic is having, they discovered they are not adequately addressing the scale of their problem. The journey on how the Aravind Eye Hospitals and Clinics address their scale opportunity will continue in our chapter on Scaling.

Challenge: start Sensing

Remember the topic, frustration or opportunity you identified in Chapter 2? This is what we call the challenge and now is the time to get to work on it. The rest of this chapter takes you through several practical practices that help you to Sense on the challenge you chose. We call these practices tools.

Tool 1: Passion and Purpose

We use Passion and Purpose during the Sensing phase when we want to tap into intrinsic motivations to discover what you can personally bring to the entrepreneurial topic at hand.

Instead of starting with *what*, start with *why*. Focus on *why* you're doing what you're doing. Focusing on *why* provides rich insights as every team member has different and personal reasons for being motivated about the topic at hand. The *why* captures the entrepreneur's inner thoughts early on, and allows you to identify with, connect with and cement your dedication to the topic that you're working on; it's your drive, your whole reason for pursuing an entrepreneurial approach to health care in the first place. Your *why* helps you, the health entrepreneur, articulate and discover why this topic really intrigues you. What matters to you individually? And then you come together as a team and find out there are lots of different motivations for entrepreneurially addressing a shared health care challenge.

Practical example

Imagine a nutritionist working in a hospital setting. Her challenge is to get patients to eat more fruit and vegetables. She thinks about her *why* and realizes that she grew up next to a farm and has amazing memories of eating fresh fruit and vegetables. She knows that if she could get other people to understand how delicious fresh produce tastes and how valuable it is for human health, then increased consumption may result. That's her *why*.

Call to action

In your team, discuss for each individual what elements of the topic are exciting to them and why. Be sure to postpone your judgment and really listen as to how everyone's reasons might be slightly different.

Tool 2: Wild Safari

Health professionals may think we know what the user experience is, but until we take time to observe users like patients, family and even co-workers, we really don't know. To be a successful health entrepreneur, we need to break away from as many second-party points of view as possible.

The Wild Safari tool compliments traditional computer research by generating insights through first-hand observation. Wild Safari is about exploring what users are doing, what they are not doing and developing an understanding of user quirks, habits, rituals and goals. Do not let this process be filtered or interpreted by what people are saying through secondhand perspectives, like market research or focus groups. Instead, collect inspiration and memorable images of what you directly observe through users.

The essence of the Wild Safari is to go out and conduct first-hand user observation in places where users are in their natural habitats to gain an understanding and empathy of what user needs are. Go to where your users spend time living, working, healing, recovering, hurting, testing, etc. Indulge your curiosity while being respectful of user privacy. Don't judge, don't interpret, just use a child's eye to observe. Take a notepad, take a pen, take a camera and capture what you see. This experience will help you get a sense of what's the norm, and what the outliers might be. Look for trends and weak signals, and zoom in on those aspects that make you question what's going on. This process will additionally help you develop empathy for the user.

Once you've collected observations, notes, photos and other documentation, reflect on what you've seen, what you've discovered, and capture the most surprising insights and user needs from your Wild Safari experience.

Pointers:

1. *Opposites:* Observe the exact opposite of what you are studying. For example, when solving the

problem of excessive waiting lines in certain parts of a hospital, look also at highly successful parts where there are barely any waiting lines.

2. *Eyes of a child:* Pretend you are a child, particularly if you are familiar with the topic at hand. Share out loud what you observe, and do the same with different partners, asking other individuals for fresh perspective from the eyes of a child. Different people will have varied observations. Person A observes for person B, person B writes person A's observations as told and vice versa.

3. *Extreme users:* Focus on extreme users, people who are really experienced or completely novice in a particular activity. Observe and note how they behave differently from regular users. For example, in a CAT scan facility, observe both people who have undergone a CAT scan many times and first-timers. How do they prepare, how do they dress, move through the room and onto the table, interact with staff? What shortcuts do or don't they take? What do they struggle with?

4. *Work-arounds:* Observe and look for shortcuts and work-arounds that users have adopted to get something done that is otherwise difficult or inconvenient. This strategy contains valuable clues for innovation – sometimes users have created a new way of doing things that points toward a clear need or a crude version of a possible innovative idea. For example, experienced patients often request specific days or times for treatment or visits because they know these times give them an advantage (e.g. shorter waiting times).

Practical example

Continuing with the eating more fruit and vegetables example, the nutritionist got up from behind her desk where she traditionally provides patient consultation. She went to a patient recovery room instead. There, in the hospital, as she was thinking about why people don't eat enough healthy food, a trolley came past the patient room full of sweets and crisps and sugary drinks. Suddenly there was this moment, this sort of "Wow, this a completely counterproductive system. Why is it still like this?" At the end of the day, the nutritionist went to pick up her kids from school where she observed chips, sugary drinks and pizzas being offered for lunch in the cafeteria. Later, the nutritionist went to the supermarket to shop for groceries and watched purchase patterns at the checkout.

Call to action

Take yourself or your team, go out to where your users are, spend at least an hour and a half observing and see what you find. Document, document, document and share what you learnt (insights and user needs) when you return. Remember to have patience and cherish the not knowing, as urgency will not help you learn more.

Tool 3: Facts and Figures

We use the Facts and Figures tool during the Sensing phase when we doubt the reliability of assumptions, and seek to discover patterns, trends and cycles from a broad set of data.

This opportunity is ideal to overthrow typical biases based on other insufficient or nonrepresentative facts. The key to Facts and Figures is pattern recognition. You're looking for an outlier that allows you to dive deeply into a world that you didn't think existed. What you're doing is collecting data to dispel myths. You're looking to discover surprise opportunities and places to investigate further. You're surfacing any weak signals that may not arise at first glance but become glaring or at least interesting with Facts and Figures.

The rationale for using the Facts and Figures tool is to:

1. Overthrow typical biases of others based on insufficient or nonrepresentative facts or faulty patterns.
2. Facilitate opportunity Sensing: allow for sizing, analysis of causality, pattern recognition, extrapolation into the future.
3. Trigger entrepreneurial ideas by studying data.

Pointers:

First, create a fact pack:

- Make a list of the different perspectives to the problem to provide direction to the research.
- Through research, compile a volume of rich data-driven visuals from various sources.
- Make the pages easy to review, use infographics, charts, tables, not paragraphs of text.
- Look for data that allows free interpretation, such as consumer blogs, instead of solely depending on traditional consumer research.

- Compile as many pages as you can of rich, data-driven visuals from infographics, charts, tables.

Then, browse through the data with a keen eye for weak signals, contradictions and surprises. Remember not to fall into the trap of the confirmation bias that was mentioned in the mind-sets part of this chapter.

Finally, draw inferences from your findings. Avoid "analysis paralysis" (i.e. overanalyzing to the point that you freeze) and capture the most surprising insights. These insights go onto your Sensing canvas.

Practical example

Back to our nutritionist example. When the nutritionist searches for ways to get people to eat more fruit and vegetables, she might review an industry report showing that only 10% of all receipts are for fresh produce. When the nutritionist looks more closely, she may notice that there's three types of produce that are selling more than others. What are they? Why would that be? She needs to go beyond the obvious and dive deeper into the numbers.

Entrepreneurship in action: data analytics at the psychiatric ward

The psychiatric ward of the University Medical Center in Utrecht (The Netherlands), was exploring the power of "big data" and new ways of analyzing data. They started with a small team

(continued)

(continued)

of data scientists and a large set of data that was stripped of patient details (anonymized). Every week, the team organized "Data Wednesday." Data Wednesday is effectively a structured Sensing moment where data scientists invite nurses and psychiatrists to ask questions and collaborate to find answers. Many questions that the nurses and psychiatrists asked were about predicting patient aggression and thus reducing risks for other patients and staff.

The analysts tried to analyze whether there were specific moments in time that were more risk prone. While they found quite a few, most were identified as not relevant, outliers or misinterpreted data by nurses and psychiatrists. A first learning from this case is that it can pay off to collaborate with experts to ensure you understand the context of certain insights before leaping to conclusions.

One moment, however, did stand out: 12pm to 1pm was identified as a clear time in the day that was prone to aggressive incidents. When the nurses and psychiatrists saw this, they quite quickly understood that lunchtime was the culprit. But why? This made them examine the lunch setup which was with all patients around one big table. They have since changed from one big table to multiple smaller tables. While they are waiting for enough data to validate this test, staff are optimistic about its results. The second learning from this case is that often data shows us insights that in hindsight are quite simple and clear (e.g. all patients together on one table at the same time creates an environment prone to aggression) but that few have seen clearly and convincingly before.

Call to action

Go ahead, give Facts and Figures a try. Alone or, preferably, in your team, create a fact pack. Spend at least an hour deeply diving into the data. What did you learn? Capture these insights. Remember to challenge your confirmation bias and be truly open to new insights.

Tool 4: User Interview + Expert Interview

The User Interview is a tool that familiarizes you with the problem from the user's viewpoint and discerns what the user has to say about the challenge at hand. Your goal is to learn how the user feels and understand the user's underlying motives. User Interview enables you to zoom in on the user experiences, issues and questions, giving you the opportunity to listen for underlying rationale, motivations and user needs or concerns.

The effectiveness of the User Interview depends on your ability to earn the trust of the user so that, together, you help articulate and explore their needs. One of the ways to earn trust is to explain your intent up front – be honest and transparent with the user about why you're asking questions. Be open with your questions. Avoid making assumptions in how you phrase your questions; focus on asking open-ended questions (i.e. questions that begin with words like "who", "what", "when", "where", "why"). Study the user's body language and listen beyond their words to appreciate emotions users may share during the User Interview. Further earn user trust by taking the user seriously and acknowledging user emotions. Once again, hold back any judgment.

As tempting as it may be, don't sympathize. Sympathy can bias interview results. Focus on staying engaged. Ask consecutive "why" questions to uncover underlying rationale, beliefs and pain points that the user may have. Why questions will help you capture surprising and contradictory user needs.

Pointers:

1. List all assumptions you have about the topic and the interview so you can park them before your interview.
2. Explain your intent. Be honest and transparent.
3. Ask diverse questions, which tend to be open questions exploring facts, emotions, the past/problem and the future/solution.
4. Attend to the whole person by listening to words as well as observing body language and emotions.
5. Earn trust by taking the user seriously. Acknowledge emotions and hold back judgment. Do not sympathize or you will bias interview results.
6. Ask several consecutive WHY questions in a row to uncover underlying rationale, beliefs and pain points. For example, if a patient says, "I do not enjoy eating vegetables," the nutritionist would ask "Why?" The patient might respond, "I don't like

the way they taste," to which the nutritionist would respond, "Why?" The patient could respond, "I don't know how to prepare vegetables properly to eat so that they taste good." The nutritionist would ask, "Why?" The patient would respond, "I grew up in a home where we ate canned or frozen vegetables." And on from there.

7. Capture the most interesting user needs and add them to your Sensing canvas.

Practical example

For our healthy food example, the nutritionist spoke to a friend at the cafeteria. They sat together at a table and discussed the user's motivations for buying fruit and vegetables. The interesting outcome was that although the user (patient, in this case) was motivated to eat more healthily and visited the local grocery

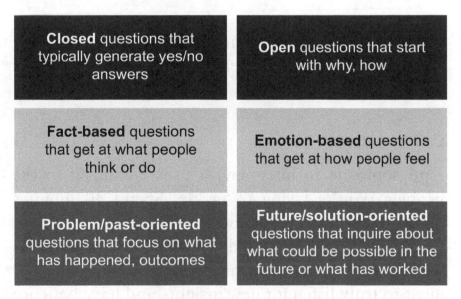

FIGURE 3.2 Types of questions

store on a regular basis, he didn't buy more than his typical three or four types of fruit. Further, during lunch at the cafeteria, there was not a single fruit on his tray. When the nutritionist asked the patient, "Why aren't you exploring the fresh fruit sold today for lunch?," the patient's answer was that the patient didn't recognize the fruit being served that day and wasn't sure he'd like the taste. Similarly, the patient explained that he doesn't know what to do with vegetables when he buys them from the supermarket. How should they be prepared? Where did they come from? What other foods should they be paired with? The nutritionist was surprised and thought,

> Hang on a second, here's someone who's trying to get healthier, wants more variety of fruit and vegetables. His hang up is not lack of choice, it's that he doesn't know what to do with vegetables once he has them.

Turns out that the patient from the User Interview is not unique in feeling challenged about vegetable preparation.

Call to action

Find someone to interview, a user entangled in the problem you're trying to tackle. Spend 30 minutes doing an in-depth interview with the user to uncover what motivates the individual. Repeat this process with multiple users. Remember to postpone your judgment to truly listen for new insights and have patience with your user.

Tool 5: User Journey

The User Journey tool helps to understand user highs and lows during a given process. We employ the User Journey to understand how a user moves through a certain course of action over a period and what he or she experiences along the way. User Journey puts a spotlight on what the user is trying to achieve by identifying interactions, objects and information that the user goes through, as well as frustrations and opportunities. What happens before a user engages in the process? What happens to the user during the process? What happens afterwards?

The important thing is to map out a time line from the beginning to the end, and identify all the activities, all the interactions your user has. What are the frustrations, opportunities and unarticulated needs of the user throughout the day? Ask or interpret what the user is trying to achieve in every action. Describe the highs and the lows of the User Journey and try to understand what's happening each step of the way.

Pointers:

1. Select the user whose journey you want to understand. Ideally, first shadow the user in his or her normal daily routines.
2. Map out a horizontal time line from beginning to end with performed activities. Stretch beginning and end beyond where most people believe it starts or ends. E.g. a visit to the GP might not start at the GP office but at the point the user feels there is a problem and might include searching the internet before contacting the GP.

3. For each activity, add:

   a. places visited;
   b. interactions with people;
   c. key objects used;
   d. information exchanged.

4. Interpret and articulate what the user's real intent is with each activity.
5. Describe the user's highs and lows. Interpret the pain points of each activity.
6. Look for and capture the most compelling user needs.

Your goal is to fully comprehend your user's needs. By documenting the user's words, actions, thoughts and feelings, you will help synthesize user clues, identify disconnects between what is said versus actions taken, as well as explore intent and drivers behind what users have said and done.

Practical example

The nutritionist mapped the shopping process that a colleague of hers goes through for their family. This process started at home reviewing a list, and continued as she went to pick up her kids and visited the grocery store. She even went home with her and joined them for dinner. Based on these interactions, she created the User Journey. Reviewing the journey with her team the day after, they noticed the frustrations in picking up the kids from school and at the grocery store and wrote these down as insights. They wondered how they might improve on this . . .

Activity	Decide on shopping list	Pick up kids from school	Buy groceries	Cook dinner	Eat dinner
Location	Home	School	Supermarket	Home	Home
Key objects used	iPhone	Car	iPhone for shopping list/shopping cart	Cooking utensils	Dishes
Information exchanged	–	Info about what's for dinner	–	–	–
Highs and lows	☺	☹ Kids often don't agree	☹ Not enough fresh, local organic produce	😐	☺

Figure 3.3 User Journey example

Call to action

Now it's your turn to go on a User Journey. Identify your user, explain what you're trying to do and follow your user for at least an hour and a half on his or her User Journey. Return and map out the experience including the moments that were highs and lows for the user. Remember to challenge your confirmation bias and take the time with your team to truly learn new things.

Tool 6: Force Fields

Force Fields enables you to zoom out to see the bigger context from a different perspective.

The Force Fields tool used during the Sensing phase focuses on the big picture, the whole system, a community within an environment that consists of interacting, interrelated and interdependent people and objects.

Force Fields looks at the factors in the value exchange, where there might be conflict and any behaviors that emerge from the whole system as it's affected by these dynamics. Force Fields can reveal important clues about motivation, intentions and needs, as well as vulnerabilities and opportunities.

The key to the Force Fields tool is to analyze the dynamics between users and stakeholders and uncover insights about the needs of users in the process. You execute this process by identifying, mapping and labelling the users, the stakeholders and any key objects in the roles that they play in the system. That exercise helps you decide what the system's boundaries are, what's included and what's not in the system. You can identify, map and label these elements within the system with different colors (we suggest different color lines) and materials and markers so that differences between material exchanges like money or immaterial dependencies like trust or recognition are visually displayed. Force Fields helps to understand prevailing dynamics and patterns in the system, and lets you take a step back to generate and capture sometimes surprising insights.

Practical example

Our nutritionist started mapping the ecosystem of players involved in daily decisions about food and the relationships between them. See Figure 3.4 below. One of her team members remarked that children seem to form an important part of this map, given the number of arrows that convene there. They noted it down as an insight. They wondered if this would be a user group to focus on.

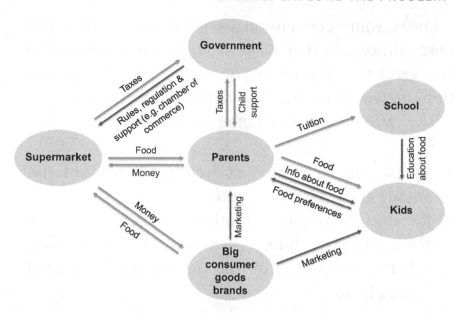

FIGURE 3.4 Force Field example

Call to action

Gather your materials and spend one hour mapping out the users, stakeholders and interactions. Then step back and see what you can glean from the Force Field and share the resulting insights on your Sensing canvas. Remember to cherish the not knowing when using this tool.

Tool 7: Reframing

Reframing (Benammar, 2012) is a powerful tool to use when you need to think differently about a topic. Perhaps there's a situation that you encounter every day that you want to approach with new perspective; Reframing can disarm skeptics by helping expose conventional wisdom that is a barrier to progress. Reframing allows you to completely flip an idea or conventional wisdom on its head.

Overturning conventional wisdom can lead to new possibilities, and that's a key to Reframing. Reframing is a great tool for when you want to shake up your thinking and push the boundaries of innovation.

The rationale for Reframing is that it:

1. Helps you to expose conventional wisdom that stands in the way of progress.
2. Exploits the inability of others to think differently; the contrarian thinker sees new directions where others are blinded by the dominant, yet unchallenged logic.
3. Trains your thinking to look at problems in fresh, unexpected ways to open new solution spaces for new ideas.

Why do people believe in a certain way of doing things or a certain way of looking at the world? Reframing entails flipping each of these supporting beliefs upside down and creating opposites for each belief. Start with a grammatical opposite. Get started by playing with words and see what comes out. Put your logic and your realism to one side to explore. Now, imagine you reframe a core belief that depicts a world in which all four overturned supporting beliefs are true. You then have a "what if" question for each of these beliefs. Use that output to stretch your thinking, and you can then use it to formulate your Creative Question.

Reframing is a conceptual direction to think out of the box, as well as a practical tool. Conceptually Reframing means allowing the underlying beliefs commonly accepted within health care to surface, and to turn these beliefs around to innovate. Tesla challenged and overturned the common belief that electric cars would have a very limited range. Green energy – cogeneration, solar and wind – overturned the common belief that only large scale centralized electric power production would be economically viable. Amazon turned the common belief that people couldn't be coaxed away from the retail experience on its head. And Apple iTunes completely toppled the common belief that one could not make money from music online.

Reframing as a practical tool is surprisingly powerful. It starts with identifying a core *limiting* belief that is relevant within your domain or industry, in this case, health care.

There is a joke about two fish that are met by a duck as they are swimming about. The duck says, "Nice water, isn't it?" When he is gone, the one fish asks the other, "What is water?" It is hard to see the thinking that you are currently immersed in. The box that limits your creativity is difficult to recognize when you have never moved outside of it. The takeaway here is to get outside of health care to explore how other industries embrace entrepreneurship. Then borrow what you learn in a way that can be applied entrepreneurially to help people in health care.

Pointers:

Reframing is not something that our fight-flight-prone, pattern-recognizing brain is good at. But you can do it using four simple steps:

49

1. Formulate and pick a strongly held core belief – a sacred cow, an obstacle, a cliché.
2. Brainstorm supporting beliefs – why do people believe this? Pick the four most intriguing ones.
3. Overturn each supporting belief: first start with the grammatical opposite; then play with words to make variations; finally make it extreme. Logic is not your friend here; the more radical or funny it is, the better. Then, select the most fun or extreme opposite for each supporting belief.
4. Now imagine a reframed core belief that describes a world in which all four selected opposites are true – "what if . . ."?

Practical example

Let's go back to our example of trying to get people to eat more fruit and vegetables. How should our nutritionist reframe in this instance? We could think about the health reality that we need to go through – the effort of cleaning, peeling and preparing our daily servings – and then use Reframing to challenge that idea. The core belief could be stated as eating fruit and vegetables is tedious and cumbersome. After going through the Reframing steps, the reframed core belief could be that there are copious ways to consume fruit and vegetables with zero effort. This type of thinking has led to product innovation in the kinds of juices, smoothies, powders, vitamins we see on the market.

Call to action

Great news: there's an online tool you can use to reframe. Go to reframe.thnk.org and spend 40 minutes

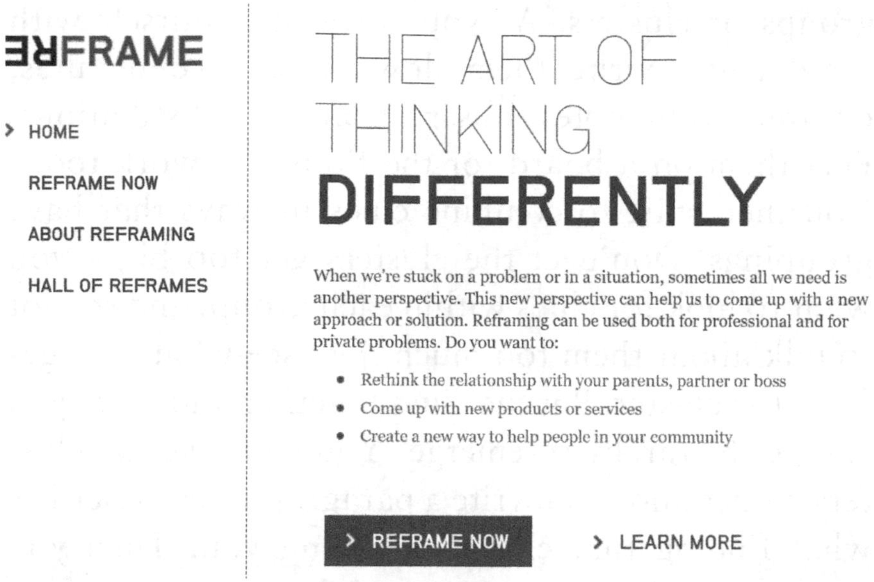

ЭЯFRAME

> HOME

REFRAME NOW

ABOUT REFRAMING

HALL OF REFRAMES

THE ART OF THINKING DIFFERENTLY

When we're stuck on a problem or in a situation, sometimes all we need is another perspective. This new perspective can help us to come up with a new approach or solution. Reframing can be used both for professional and for private problems. Do you want to:

- Rethink the relationship with your parents, partner or boss
- Come up with new products or services
- Create a new way to help people in your community

> REFRAME NOW   > LEARN MORE

FIGURE 3.5 Online Reframing tool

Reframing. Remember to postpone your judgment. Particularly with this tool, your judgment can get in the way of going out of the box and seeing new realities.

Tool 8: Connecting the Dots

Throughout Sensing, you've gathered a variety of user needs and insights. Now you want to see the bigger picture, and you want this picture to fit on one page.

Connecting the Dots is a tool that helps round out the Sensing phase by helping to identify new relationships between the clues and to find meaning from those clues. Connecting the Dots allows you to get new themes and insights, and even lets new user needs emerge. The result is a bigger picture view of the Sensing work that you've completed to date.

Connecting the Dots is a clustering process. Take every piece of information you've gathered and form groups or clusters. As you surround yourself with these clues, write them down and take pictures, organize your notes, observations and distillations. Post them on a board (or the floor can work too!). You then start to combine clues in ways that have groupings. Don't let the clusters get too big – you want to look for clues within each group, and try not to talk about them too much, just see what emerges from the cluster. Put the clues together and see if you can get hierarchy to emerge. You can give the clusters names and even write a paragraph that describes what finding that cluster is telling you. Then you can get together as a group and discuss outcomes to agree on the most intriguing and emergent clusters that you can leverage for your Creative Question.

Practical example

In the nutritionist's healthy food project, she found lots of information and insights about eating and drinking habits in schools, hospitals, the workplace and at home. But it is the overlap between these food habits that the nutritionist wants to cluster. The overlapping theme that emerges from the Sensing process is that consuming food is largely about convenience for most people. Also, there seems to be a cluster around children and schools that seems to be a point of frustration as well as an opportunity for solutions.

Call to action

With your team, print and take in all the user needs, insights and imagery you've gathered. Arrange it on a board so that it's easy to view the big picture. Use 30 minutes to cluster this data before moving on to the Creative Question.

Tool 9: Creative Question

The Creative Question is the end of the Sensing phase. It helps you get to the crux of the problem that needs to be solved. The Creative Question allows you to generate new ideas and can help you disrupt the way you looked at your original thinking.

By formulating a Creative Question, you can get new findings from the whole of your Sensing experience, which ultimately helps you articulate a more relevant way to look at the original problem. Your Creative Question should connect to your Passion and Purpose. Your Creative Question provides direction and paints a whole new solution space from which you can generate more ideas.

Your Creative Question will help you narrow, broaden or deepen the original concept you explored into compelling questions that beg to be answered. A Creative Question should start with the words "How might we." Research suggests that this formulation harnesses most creative power; the words allow for more dreaming and more diverse ideas than "How can we," for example. How do you form your Creative Question? You do so by focusing on clusters of insight, user needs and inspirations. You must keep iterating until you have a strong question that can launch you into Visioning (the next phase after Sensing).

Entrepreneurship in action: Creative Question for a Philips CT scan

A health specialist from Philips was given the task of upgrading a CT scan (sometimes known as a CAT scan) facility of a children's hospital. Together with a leading radiologist in the hospital they started Sensing by observing and interviewing children, child psychologists and hospital staff to try to uncover a bigger picture. In Sensing, they uncovered that children experience fear, anxiety, feeling sick, boredom and loneliness resulting in them not lying still enough for the scan or not even wanting to get in the scan in the first place. This often means either the scan has to be repeated, with the inevitable second dose of radiation and additional costs, or they have to be sedated, which is even more distressing for both child and family, and can add four hours to the total time involved in the scan procedure.

Additional Sensing work gave them more insights. First, children associate memories strongly with locations – so a bad experience during a scan procedure will mean they do not want to go back there. Children will respond positively if they are given influence over their procedure. And finally, storytelling is a powerful way of engaging children, and can provide positive distraction during medical procedures.

This allowed the team to create a powerful Creative Question: how might we give children an amazing experience while undergoing a cat scan? This question is bold (amazing experience and cat scan), has the user at its center and is exciting to answer. Most importantly, it allowed the team to come up with a very innovative way to solve the problem.

The new CAT scan experience starts with storytelling around a character selected by the child – like a dolphin or an elephant. This character is a little ill, so the child is able to perform a mini CAT scan, the so-called Kitten scanner, to find out why this character is not feeling well. This gives the child insight and empathy into what they are about to encounter themselves.

When the child enters the scan room, the ambience of the room changes to the character preference of the child, providing an engaging environment through lighting, sounds and animations, which continues the storytelling in the preparation room. The animation is synchronized with the medical procedure, including friendly instructions at important moments in the scan, such as "hold your breath until the elephant's trunk is full."

This project, and countless since, is a big success. First-time-right treatments have increased, sedation rates have dropped and, as a result, additional radiation doses have been avoided. The efficiency of use for the scanner facility has increased, which reduces costs for the hospital and the health care system in general, and most importantly, the quality of the experience for all parties went up.

Pointers:

1. Formulate a Creative Question for a user, based on intriguing insights and user needs. Use this formula: how might we [HMW] [Action Verb] for a [User] with [Need], given that they [Insight]. E.g. HMW create a better MRI experience for kids who need to be comforted, given that they have already started to be scared at home before they visit the hospital.

2. Aim to "have your cake and eat it too": find the right level of tension or paradox for the Creative Question to stimulate your creativity. E.g. HMW create for kids a better pre- and in-hospital MRI experience that they will enjoy.

3. Take an unreasonable stance to stimulate radical rather than incremental innovation. E.g. how might we give kids the best MRI hospital experience that they will love!

4. Pick the right level of abstraction for the Creative Question: don't boil the ocean, don't boil an egg. Ask "what" if too abstract, ask "why" if too concrete. Too abstract: how might we redesign the hospital? Too concrete: how might we improve the lying position in the MRI machine? Just right: how might we redesign the MRI experience to be enjoyable.

5. Make sure not to include a solution in the Creative Question. E.g. "how might we prepare kids at home to make the MRI experience fun?" is better than "how might we create a comic book to prepare kids for undergoing an MRI?"

Practical example

The nutritionist and her team got very excited about the opportunity to focus on schools and children as a way to influence the system. They formulated their Creative Question as: how might we use schools to make fruit and vegetable consumption convenient and fun?

Call to action

Take 30 minutes with your team to sit down and draft a Creative Question that's going to kick-start a whole new landscape for ideas.

Chapter 4

Visioning

We're in the Visioning phase (the second phase of the Innovation Flow), which means you ideate many new concepts with team members and then cluster and select to settle on one. Visioning is centered around imagining new concepts and ideas based on the Creative Question you developed in the Sensing phase. The more ideas you generate during the Visioning phase, the better. This chapter guides your entrepreneurial journey as you:

- diverge and create many new ideas;
- go through various ideation techniques;
- combine existing ideas in a new context;
- converge to select the ideas that are most exciting.

At the end of this Visioning chapter, you will understand the concept of Visioning, you will have explored the required mind-sets and you will have worked on your challenge with tools from the Visioning tool kit (Hilberts, 2018). We will conclude this chapter by an idea that you will take forward in the next step of your entrepreneurial journey: Prototyping.

Introduction to Visioning

Visioning (Nooyen et al., 2014) – the process of coming up with breakthrough ideas – is often assumed to be an isolated and instantaneous affair. We have images of the isolated creative genius experiencing a moment of *eureka!* in the bathtub, or a great vision while fasting in the desert. What commonly happens is that a new concept is developed over a sustained time. Looking back, such a period will be riddled with moments of serendipity, moments where lucky connections, unexpected insights and breakthroughs made the difference. These breakthroughs are rarely the product of one mind; they are almost always the result of cross-pollination of ideas, and approaches from a different field being applied to the field the creative person is working in. For example, Gutenberg, in 1450, combined insights from wine-pressing and his profession as a goldsmith to create a printing system that led to the first assembly-line-style mass production of books (Giges, 2012).

Visioning is a phase that consists of two parts: first, the divergent part where we generate many ideas and second the convergent part where we combine, cluster and select to end up with one idea or solution. The divergent part of Visioning is about quantity more than quality. It's widely assumed that there's a trade-off between quantity and quality – if you want to do better work, you must do less of it – but this turns out to be false. In fact, when it comes to idea generation, quantity is the most predictable path to quality. So how do we maximize our odds of creating a truly great new insight, and a valuable concept? We come up with many ideas. On average, creative geniuses aren't qualitatively better in their fields than their peers. They simply produce a greater volume of work, which gives them more variation and a higher chance of originality. Edison famously said he found 1,000 ways not to make a lightbulb before he found the one way that did (Elkhorne, 1967). Many people fail to achieve true originality because they generate only a few ideas and then obsess about refining them to perfection. How many clinicians do you know who aim at refining as opposed to perfection?

Divergent vs. convergent thinking

Divergent thinking involves creative methods to generate multiple answers to a set question. Key words that represent divergence are broadening, alternatives, quantity, co-creation, dialogue, chaos, intuition. Convergent thinking involves aiming for a single, correct solution to a problem. Key words include focusing, selecting, quality, choices, discussion, grip, structure, logic.

The process of Visioning may seem both daunting and mysterious. Indeed, it is in no way straightforward. An understanding of what's entailed in a structured Visioning process will create better results for Visioning to be successful. Engaging with other people to work and interact in an open, connected network, significantly increases the chance of these "lucky" moments (Johnson, 2010). We know that being an

Diverging	Converging
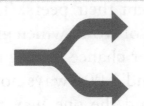	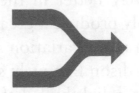
• Going for volume	• Going for quality
• Generating	• Selective
• Supporting	• Criticizing
• Yes and …	• Yes but …

FIGURE 4.1 Diverging versus converging

extravert does not correlate with being creative, but being connected does. According to Steven Johnson's work, *Where Good Ideas Come From* is what happened in 18th century coffeehouses in Europe: these spaces allowed different perspectives, experiences and areas of expertise to connect, which created a fertile environment for innovation, which for one thing led to the period of Enlightenment (Johnson, 2010).

Breakthrough ideas are rarely the product of one mind. They are almost always the result of a cross-pollination of ideas and approaches. For instance, no editorial staff could ever outperform the knowledge of the crowd, hence *Wikipedia* replaced *Encyclopedia Britannica*.

Entrepreneurship is a nonlinear path, not a straight one. Entrepreneurship often feels like two steps forward and one step back, sometimes even more steps back. Other times the process of entrepreneurship, especially in the Visioning phase, includes jumps rather than steps that lead to a different direction altogether compared to what you'd originally intended. The process invariably has moments of frustration as the initial challenge frame can prove too constraining or preliminary entrepreneurial explorations offer less impressive results than hoped for. Successful Visioning has core characteristics. Your job is to create as many of these conditions as possible. This book advocates for trying to systematically explore entrepreneurship in the context of health care. Below are a few suggestions to navigate the Visioning process.

A major challenge before you that's part of the Visioning process is to combine existing bits of information with new insights and new interpretations of the world to address a health care need. To do so, explore a "slow hunch" – this suggestion is especially relevant in health care because human life is involved. A slow hunch is the feeling an innovative idea or vision is to be found in a certain direction without being able to pinpoint it yet. By pursuing this hunch, over time, the idea crystallizes. It becomes clearer and clearer. Even though Charles Darwin himself claimed the theory of natural selection occurred to him on September 28, 1838, while reading Thomas Malthus's essay on population, Darwin's own notebooks reveal that the theory was forming clearly in his mind more than a year before: it wasn't a flash of insight, but what Steven Johnson calls a "slow hunch."

Rice University professor Erik Dane found that the more expertise and experience people gain, the more entrenched they become in a particular way of viewing the world. That reality is particularly

(continued)

(continued)

frightening for health entrepreneurship given the duration of training required for health personnel. How do we maintain an entrepreneurial mind-set? The unique combination of deep experience and broad interest is critical. Health entrepreneurs embrace the tendency to seek novelty and variety in intellectual, aesthetic and emotional pursuits. A representative study of thousands of Americans showed that both entrepreneurs and inventors were more likely than their peers to have leisure time hobbies that involved drawing, painting, architecture, sculpture and literature (Eschleman et al., 2014). Highly creative adults moved to new cities more frequently than their peers during their childhood, which gave them exposure to different cultures and values, and encouraged flexibility and adaptability. Living abroad didn't matter: it was time *immersing* abroad. The more the foreign culture differed from their native one, the more that experience contributed to their creativity. The third and most important factor was depth – the amount of time spent working abroad. Short stints did little good.

Visioning is not forecasting. Forecasting is predicting what will happen, whereas Visioning is ultimately about *making* it happen. Successful entrepreneurship in health care means having such a strong conviction that an idea will work, that its realization is driven with relentless commitment, ultimately saving human lives.

This compulsive determination is required to push through all the barriers and convince the critics.

> Our judgment is most accurate in domains where we have a lot of experience and where we can make predictions. In environments that are changing or unpredictable, we risk being overconfident. The more successful people have been in the past, the worse they perform when they enter a new environment. They are less likely to seek critical feedback even though the context is radically different. Nonexperts – which include "experts" in environments that are rapidly changing – make sounder judgments when they conduct a thorough analysis.

Visioning brings the backgrounds, attitudes, emotions and dynamics of the creative team and of each individual team member involved to the equation. Health care is especially ripe for entrepreneurial breakthroughs due to the rich diversity of health care professionals, among other reasons. Choice of team members matters enormously. Ask yourself, would I want to be stuck with that team member during a tough situation? Would I want to work for that person one day? (Rich, 2016).

Note that introverts ideate differently than extroverts. Facilitate a healthy Visioning process by giving space to both introverts and extroverts. Let team members write ideas first to get them out of their heads before the team jumps into group brainstorming.

Success cannot be ensured. Any attempt at creative leadership to realize a big vision or a breakthrough concept is risky – the probability of failure or disappointment is very significant. The rule of thumb of venture capital firms is that in their portfolio maybe one out of ten will become the huge success, while the large majority just survive or flounder and must be closed. So, the idea is to strive for a truly great outcome, do everything possible to make it happen, but realize that the probability of a huge success is small and therefore adapt constantly to new insights and opportunities.

It's okay to be afraid

Being a health entrepreneur entails taking the "road less traveled" by clinicians, championing a novel approach or set of ideas to improve health care (Frost, 1916). It involves introducing and advancing an idea that's relatively unusual within health care with the potential to improve it. Health entrepreneurs are people who take the initiative to make their visions a reality for the betterment of our community. It's okay to feel fear and doubt – it'd be weird if you didn't experience those feelings. What sets health entrepreneurs apart is that you act despite your fear. You know in your heart that failing would yield less regret than failing to try. Your patients' lives and well-being are at stake.

The Visioning mind-sets

How many times have we thought to ourselves or heard people say, "I want to be an entrepreneur" or "I want to run my own business, but I don't have the idea. I am waiting for the idea to come to me." Not knowing when you are going to get that breakthrough idea is what makes entrepreneurship both fun and frustrating. The following mind-sets should help you get there faster.

> Not knowing when you are going to get that breakthrough idea is what makes creativity equally magical and frustrating.

Yes and . . .

The divergent part of Visioning is primarily a social process. You cannot really brainstorm alone and often one person just has half an idea that only becomes good if it's combined with another person's idea. To make this collaboration successful, it's key to not challenge or dismiss ideas of others. Rather encourage people by acknowledging all ideas (even the craziest) and by building on them. In other words: always say "Yes and . . ." rather than "Yes but . . ."

Go for volume

The Nobel Prize-winning chemist Linus Pauling once said, "If you want to have good ideas you must have many ideas. Most of them will be wrong, and what you have to learn is which ones to throw away." If you find yourself worrying that it is hard to tell between the bad ones and the good ones, don't worry: you are still warming up and your best ideas have yet to come. Don't be too judgmental on yourself but just stick with it.

Go for multiple waves

As your mind works hard to find more innovative ideas, you will reach a point where you feel you (or your team) have hit a brick wall and you can't think of anything else. This is when self-doubt and defeat can often creep in. You feel that your ideas will never crystallize. What's really happening is you're entering the dark tunnel, the bottom of the U, a temporary space without inspiration. It's truly temporary, the tunnel will end, the U will go up again and there will be a next wave of inspiration. Even more importantly, following waves are typically more interesting than earlier waves. This is often where the real good stuff comes.

Leverage the slow bake

We typically do our Visioning in pressure cooker brainstorming sessions: time-bound moments in which the ideas should come. While this is a really strong way to generate volume, don't forget to allow for slower processes. During the entire process of gathering information and thinking of ideas, you have also been feeding your unconscious. If your unconscious mind sees that the conscious mind is determined and passionate about finding a creative breakthrough, it will deem it worthy of putting its processing power behind it. It's important to remember that your unconscious will assume the subject is not worth it if the hard conscious work has not been put in.

There's one good reason why you want your unconscious involved. It processes data 500,000 times faster than your conscious mind (Pavitt, 2016).

What's important at this stage of Visioning is not to get too stressed. You're entering the uncontrolled part of the process and this is where you must be patient. Of course, you shouldn't totally zone out doing something mindless, such as watching TV or checking up on Facebook. It's like a pot left to simmer: you don't need to stand over watching it, but at the same time you can't go out and leave it unattended.

The writer Hilary Mantel advised to remain patient:

> If you get stuck, get away from your desk. Take a walk, take a bath, go to sleep, make a pie, draw, listen to music, meditate, and exercise. Whatever you do, don't just stick there scowling at the problem. But don't make telephone calls or go to a party – if you do, other people's words will pour in where your lost words should be. Open a gap for them, create a space.
>
> (Mantel, 2010)

The feeling is like being stuck on a crossword puzzle clue. You're sure you know the answer and it's on the tip of your tongue, but you just can't think of what it is. Frustrated, you give up and go and make a cup of coffee. Just as you're stirring the coffee, the answer comes to you as if from nowhere.

The moment of insight to your problem will often come when you are doing a mundane and repetitive activity. How often have you heard people say, "I get my best ideas when I'm walking or driving home from work, having a shower, or doing the dishes"? There's a reason for this: while you're doing these simple activities, your controlled thinking takes its foot off the gas, making room for your uncontrolled thinking and allowing your mind to wander.

Give patience a chance

Health care professionals are just as entrepreneurial whether they walk inside on a treadmill or are outside in the fresh air, so it's not about the inspiring surroundings. The secret lies in the mundane physical activity that lets the prefrontal cortex take a back seat, letting your mind wander.

As the painter Joan Miró said, "I work better when I am not working than when I am" (Miró & Lubar, 1964).

We have two modes of thinking: the first is the cognitive control network, which creates focused, controlled thinking. At the heart of controlled thinking is the prefrontal cortex, the home of most of our conscious thoughts. The second is the default mode network. This mode is linked with mind wandering, (day) dreaming, free association and linking to messages we unconsciously think about.

The default mode network (uncontrolled thought) is triggered when the prefrontal cortex shuts down or relaxes. The most obvious example of this is dreams. When we are asleep, so is our prefrontal cortex (Pavitt, 2018).

Dreams have helped people find solutions to problems in the arts, science and business. A dream gave Mary Shelley the idea for *Frankenstein*, Paul McCartney the music for "Yesterday", August Kekule the shape of the Benzene molecule, Elias Howe how a sewing machine would work, and Larry Page dreamt of downloading the entire Web. Not satisfied with this achievement, Page also had the idea for the Google PageRank by dreaming of the links between the pages.

Unfortunately, we risk not capturing the ideas when we come up with creative solutions in our dreams. Being half asleep relaxes the control of the prefrontal cortex, allowing us access to the uncontrolled power of the default mode network while still being aware enough to capture what emerges. Hypnagogia is the transitional state between wakefulness and sleep. Both states – which occur in the early morning stages of not being fully awake yet and the last moment at night when you are about to drop off to sleep – are strong times for interesting ideas to arise. Edison famously tried to tap into this "Twilight Zone" with metal balls: he would sit upright in a chair and take a nap while holding a large metal ball in each hand. Once asleep, the balls would drop out of his hands and startle him awake, and he would immediately write down what was in his mind at the time.

Activities that help the prefrontal cortex to relax can also have a very beneficial effect. This is why mundane activities are so good for triggering moments of creative insight, for instance while doing the dishes, walking, taking a shower and driving home from work. Einstein would work hard on a problem for a couple of hours and then stop to play the violin (Clark, 1971). Playing a piece he knew well would require little conscious effort allowing his mind to wander and ideas to arise. By his account, "The theory of relativity occurred to me by intuition, and music is the driving force behind this intuition."

Another powerful way to nurture creative thinking is by walking. Many of history's great creatives knew this, including Beethoven, Tchaikovsky, Lucian Freud, John Milton, and Charles Dickens and Darwin. Steve Jobs was famous for holding meetings while he was walking and Mark Zuckerberg is now following in his footsteps (Umoh, 2018).

Dr. Marily Oppezzo and Daniel Schwartz, professors at Stanford University, have compared the levels of creativity in people while walking and sitting. Their research showed that their creative output increased by 60% when people walk (Oppezzo & Schwartz, 2014).

Entrepreneurship in action: the Aravind Eye Hospitals and Clinics

"If Coca-Cola can sell billions of sodas and McDonald's can sell billions of burgers," asks Dr. Venkataswamy (Dr. V), "why can't Aravind sell millions of sight-restoring operations, and, eventually, the belief in human perfection?" (www.fastcompany.com/675800/and-then-theres-dr-v).

As we learned in reading the previous chapters, the Aravind Eye Hospitals and Clinics in India revolutionized the entire system of providing eye surgeries with astonishing results both in financial terms and in terms of health outcomes. The Aravind Eye Hospitals and Clinics in India have been helping the blind population with access to high-quality care at affordable rates. Aravind stemmed from the vision of Dr. V and his passion for caring for all.

Building from success, the outcomes stemmed from the key act of Visioning – generating a variety of solutions. The general associations between fast food and sodas with health care are related to being unhealthy. It took vision to step back and look at the model of delivery as a strong platform for providing quality eye-care. The result, US$1 eye surgery that takes ten minutes but which costs around $1,650 in the US.

From an operational standpoint, the Aravind model significantly varies from typical health care hospitals and clinics. The operations leverage engagement and technology in a way that was not historically done. The clinic focuses on creating eye-care camps that are hosted by the community for the community removing the logistical burden from caregivers. This empowers the opportunity for thousands of clinics each year, serving millions of individuals over this time, providing the gift of sight.

The financial model of Aravind rest on a model that creates only a portion of its value from its customer base. Aravind has been able to provide high-quality, low-cost services for the 50 to 60% of its patients that are not able to pay market rate by using the profits from the remaining 40 to 50% of its paying patients. The quality of the services, however, are aligned between both paying and nonpaying patients (https://rctom.hbs.org/submission/aravind-eye-care-system-mcdonaldization-of-eye-care/). This is also not a typical financial model in the health care industry. Dr. V looked outside of the traditional financial models to vision what was possible.

The divergence from both typical operational and financial models has also created a new standard for Aravind for quality metrics. The model has not deteriorated the quality, but rather the quality metrics indicate that adverse events during surgery are almost two times better than for similar surgeries in the UK.

Ultimately, the success of the Aravind hospitals and clinics was set, in part, due to the key work of Visioning. Aravind's team was able to look at the goal and challenges through a completely different lens and combine existing ideas into a completely new context. They were faced with the question of the viability of the concept and engaged others to challenge their assumptions (https://opinionator.blogs.nytimes.com/2013/01/16/in-india-leading-a-hospital-franchise-with-vision/).

Challenge: start Visioning

Now it's time to get to action. Entrepreneurship doesn't happen by reading a book but through practice and real-world action. With your team, go back to the topic you started working on. The rest of this chapter takes you through several Visioning tools that help you generate a wide range of ideas that answer your Creative Question from the previous chapter. The tools end by helping you and your team settle on the one idea that you want to move forward into Prototyping.

Tool 10: Brainsketching

During Sensing, we asked you to focus on finding user needs and insights rather than focusing on ideas. You probably found it impossible to stop your mind from coming up with ideas; it's what our mind does. Now it's time to tap into that stream of creativity.

We use the Brainsketching tool for three reasons. First, when we want to get started on new ideas this tool is ideal since it taps into what's already there. You just purge all the ideas that were already in your mind and sketch them on Post-its. We also use the tool when we want to create room for introverts – people who thrive less in group discussions and prefer time to think before they speak. That's because this tool is done in silence and individually, before sharing outcomes. Finally, Brainsketching leverages the fact that the more creative part of the brain is closely associated with thinking in images rather than words.

When using this tool, you might notice that at some point you run out of ideas. This moment can be frustrating and can trick you to move on. Try not to give up, but stick with the problem a bit longer. After a while, your brain will come up with more solutions. This is what we call a second wave. Typically, the first wave contains some of the obvious solutions; it's the second (or third or fourth) wave that contains the really good stuff.

Practical example

In our example of getting people to eat more fruit and vegetables, the nutritionist invited some colleagues to sketch answers to her Creative Question on Post-its. She gave them five minutes to sketch at least four "normal ideas" and at least four "crazy ideas." After the five minutes were up, they shared their ideas starting with the crazy ones.

Call to action

Collect your team, grab Post-its and spend at least five minutes in silence sketching ideas for your Creative Question. After that time is up, share the ideas with each other. Remember to go for volume and allow multiple waves of creativity to happen.

Tool 11: Random Force

You're in need of original ideas. How do you trick your mind (which is rational) into creating brand-new perspectives and radical ideas?

Our mind is well trained to see patterns and trends and make connections. These patterns can sometimes help us interpret our world, yet they can also stand in the way of looking at the world with a fresh lens, which is important during Visioning. The Random Force tool provokes your thinking to snap out of these established patterns. You can pair two findings that have nothing in common and take a fresh perspective, which leads to new ideas where none existed before. This process encourages you to move beyond the apprehension of thinking illogically.

The key to using the Random Force tool is that it creates a connection between two completely different ideas to spark a brand-new idea. Start with your Creative Question. Next, choose a prompt – e.g. out of a magazine or look out the window. What do you see? A tree? Sidewalk? It's okay (even good!) for the prompt to be random. Use this prompt to trigger a new train of thought. Once you've chosen the prompt, quickly agree on a few key attributes of the prompt with your team. Then, individually and silently, take five minutes to sketch or write five to six ideas about how to solve your Creative Question using the attributes of that prompt. Really crazy ideas will probably follow, which helps lead to great, solid ideas.

Practical example

In our example, the nutritionist performed the Random Force tool by first grabbing a magazine. On the first page she opened, she noticed a boat and asked, "What are the attributes of a boat?" The answers were things like: it floats, it helps people across waters, it prevents people from getting wet, it's a fun way to travel . . . She then selected one of these attributes: "it's a fun way to travel" and asked, "How might we get children to eat more fruit and vegetables by making it fun?" After coming up with ideas for a while, she moved on to another attribute e.g. "it prevents people from getting wet" and asked, "How might we prevent people from eating anything except fruit and vegetables?" One of the ideas that came up was to replace the cafeteria with a farm. While this was maybe somewhat extreme, the idea made them think: maybe we can bring the farm closer to schools . . .

Call to action

Collect your team, grab random prompts (e.g. magazines), and spend 30 minutes seeing if you can push yourself to generate new ideas for your Creative Question. Don't forget that you might sometimes run dry for a while. In that case, don't worry and stick with the problem because you know the next wave of ideas will come and will be better. Remember to go for volume, allow multiple waves of creativity to happen and build on each other by saying yes and . . . rather than yes but . . .

Tool 12: Analogies for Inspiration

The purpose of Analogies for Inspiration is to generate fresh ideas by looking at your entrepreneurial idea through different lenses. Analogies for Inspiration comes in handy when we need lots of fresh ideas and want to jump-start our inspiration. Analogies for Inspiration is provocative and can help entertain ideas that may seem patently wrong. We'll use lateral thinking skills from your right brain to generate ideas, a brief holiday from logical thinking and sequential steps.

The way Analogies for Inspiration works is that you take your Creative Question and think of a familiar context where a similar question has been tackled. Explore this analogy for the elements that made it successful and look to see if you can take those same elements to apply successfully to your Creative Question.

This process of Analogies for Inspiration will help generate new ideas that you may not have otherwise imagined or explored.

Practical example

The nutritionist asks her team what analogous situations they know for their Creative Question. One of the team members remarks that this problem is analogous to getting people to stop smoking and that one element that really helped was banning smoking from bars, restaurants and offices. This allowed the team to come up with various ideas of how to ban unhealthy foods from school canteens entirely. One of the ideas was to replace the canteen with a farmers' market.

Call to action

Get together with your team. Take 30 minutes and practice Analogies for Inspiration. Make sure you capture your new ideas on Post-its. Remember to go for volume, allow multiple waves of creativity to happen and build on each other by saying yes and . . . rather than yes but . . .

Tool 13: Idea Jackpot

The purpose of the Idea Jackpot is to trigger new ideas by mixing and matching existing ingredients. The Idea Jackpot:

- shakes up and rearranges elements of the Creative Question to challenge existing thought processes and find new answers;

- explores all possible variations of the existing bits and pieces;
- snaps existing information together into provocative new patterns.

The Idea Jackpot tool is especially useful when looking for fresh ideas and when we want to stretch our thinking. The Idea Jackpot challenges you to find new answers and solutions, and it allows you to explore even more variations of the existing bits and pieces.

Begin by focusing on your Creative Question. Agree with your team on the most critical parameters within your Creative Question, usually three to five parameters without which the core of that question would not exist. List those critical parameters horizontally, which is the jackpot row. Below each parameter, list as many variations and possible alternatives for those parameters, at least five; those alternatives are your jackpot columns. Then make random runs through the five-by-five grid and select one item from each jackpot column, combining them into entirely new forms. Through the Idea Jackpot, you're combining information together into new provocative patterns to more deeply explore your Creative Question.

Practical example

Our nutritionist used the Idea Jackpot tool to explore how to get people to eat more fruit and vegetables. The key words in her Creative Question are children, eat, fruit and vegetables. She placed these words across the top of the grid. Next, she identified variations to children like kids, women, animals, parents, teachers and friends. In the eat column she came up with words like drink, buy, snack, freeze and grow. When she looked at the fruit and vegetables column, she identified the words frozen fruit, exotic vegetables, bananas, vitamins and smoothies.

The grouping she picked was kids, drink, vitamins. This combination led the team to a whole range of ideas to add vitamins to drinks that kids already took, like milk (with cereals), sports drinks and even adding vitamins to the water fountains in schools.

Call to action

This tool has a digital version. Go to ideajackpot.thnk. org and take 30 minutes with your team to conjure up new ideas. Make sure to write each idea onto a Post-it

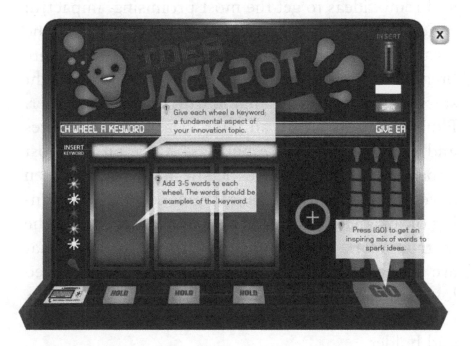

FIGURE 4.2 Online Idea Jackpot tool

so you can easily use it later. Remember to go for volume, allow multiple waves of creativity to happen and build on each other by saying yes and . . . rather than yes but . . .

Tool 14: Bright Stars and Solar Systems

Now it's time to go from quantity to quality or from diverging to converging.

We use the Bright Stars and Solar Systems tool to help filter the multitude of concepts you've generated. Bright Stars enables us to separate the good from the bad and ugly. This process yields concepts that are more likely to succeed and create breakthrough impact; it remixes and expands the best ideas for even stronger concepts to emerge.

The essence of the Bright Stars tool is to rank, pick and remix ideas to get the most promising, impactful concept. Start by creating a two-by-two matrix of the ideas that are most feasible and most likely to create breakthrough impact. Label these categories as bright stars, wild cards, low-hanging fruit and don't bother. Plot your ideas – take all your ideas on sticky notes and put them into these buckets. Agree on the most appealing ideas and where they fit in the matrix. Then develop the selected ideas into a concept by combining or expanding the ideas that are related within the matrix. Work on getting the right mix of ideas that are at once pragmatic and ambitious, add related low-hanging fruit ideas to make your big idea more realistic, or loop in wild card ideas to make it bigger and bolder.

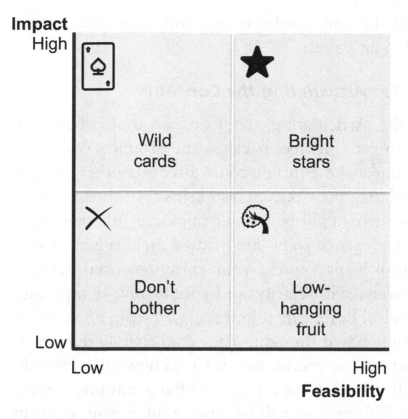

FIGURE 4.3 Bright Stars and Solar Systems grid

Practical example

In our example, the nutritionist and her team decided that "a farmers' market in every school in the city" was a bright star idea. They combined this bright star with another low-hanging fruit idea "local farmers come and showcase their fresh produce in schools and explain their origins" to create a Solar System.

Call to action

Take one hour with your team to move the Post-its with the ideas you've generated onto the Bright Stars and Solar Systems grid. Remember to leverage the slow bake and maybe revisit your selection after a good night's sleep.

Tool 15: Articulating the Concept

Use the Articulating the Concept tool when you need to get your feet back on the ground. Your goal is to make the concept come alive for other people. Articulating the Concept also helps spot the inconsistencies there might be in your thinking. Whereas other tools we've tried so far are focused on idea generation, this tool helps express your entrepreneurial concept cohesively, with clarity and specifically; it taps into the logical brain function, generates sequential, linear and time-based thought. Your challenge here is to be deliberate, use precise words to acknowledge the subtle differences in meaning and interpretation of every word. This process will help you explain your concept cohesively and precisely.

So, how to do it? Use the why, what, how framework. Start with why. Why is the idea relevant? Why is it appealing? Why does it solve the problem? Then move on to what – the essence, the alluring vision, the novel concept, the key benefits that are offered. And finally, the how – the compelling and concrete ideas to make this concept come to life. Write down every word you use to explore the why, what, how framework.

Practical example

Looking at the concept of putting a farmers' market at every school, our nutritionist works with her team to write out the concept in detail. She starts with the why: the importance of healthy eating for kids and their development and the key role schools play in facilitating this and in creating habits. The team then moves on to explaining the concept in detail including the benefits for kids, schools and parents. They finish with a description of how they would start to put this idea into practice.

Call to action

Take 30 minutes with your team to practice Articulating the Concept. Remember to build on each other by saying yes and . . . rather than yes but . . .

Tool 16: Show Me the Money

Show Me the Money explores the economic viability and the rough size of your concept in monetary terms. We need to first determine how users most benefit from your concept. What type of value do users receive from your idea? Guess how much users would be willing to pay, and how many potential users you could get interested in buying your product or service. Estimate the potential annual revenue that you could generate. Consider possible pricing and revenue models. Next, identify and ballpark the main business and societal cost components. Keep iterating until your potential income is in line with your costs and the non-monetary impact your concept generates. Now, does it seem viable enough an idea to pursue? If not, consider smart ways to increase the value received while reducing the costs. Make informed guesses at the market share your concept could realize and guesstimate the potential market size from it. Does your market share seem sizable enough to pursue? Throughout the process, keep sanity checking and adjusting these numbers as you move forward.

Show Me the Money is especially useful for when you're ready to make your entrepreneurial concept financially viable. The rationale for using Show Me the Money is that it:

- invites initial thinking about monetization of the user and social impact delivered to beneficiaries;
- provides guidance to increase the economical viability and impact of the concept;
- is a prerequisite in any further discussion with future funders of the next development stages of your entrepreneurial idea.

Show Me the Money pointers:

1. Determine how users benefit most from your concept. What type of value is created for users when using your concept (V)? Consider material (e.g. financial), immaterial (brand) and social impact value created.
2. Estimate how much people will pay for this value (P) and how many users you could get (Q). How many beneficiaries will be impacted positively (B)?
3. Estimate the potential annual revenue (=P×Q) and social impact you could generate (=B×V).
4. Identify and ballpark the main business, social and environmental cost components (C). Compare costs with revenue and impact. Iterate until your revenue and impact is much greater than all costs (P×Q)+(B×V)>C.

5. Does it seem viable enough to go after it? If not viable, consider smart ways to increase the value or benefits received while reducing the costs.

Practical example

In the challenge of trying to get people to eat more fruit and vegetables, the nutritionist and her team came up with the idea of putting farmers' markets in each school. Using this tool, they plotted the various stakeholders and the way they interacted (Figure 4.4). That led them to estimate the price parents are willing to pay, the amount of parents per school, the costs for one meal and the value created, which in this case is reduced health care costs for the beneficiaries who are the kids.

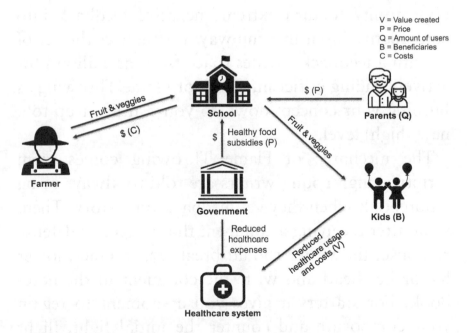

FIGURE 4.4 Show Me the Money example

Call to action

Gather with your team and spend at least an hour using the Show Me the Money tool to flush out the elements that form your business case and try to calculate V, P, Q, B and C. And see whether $(P \times Q)+(B \times V)$ is bigger than C. Remember to leverage the slow bake and maybe revisit your outcomes after a good night's sleep or a few days.

Tool 17: Flame Throwing

At this point in the entrepreneurial process, we've got our concept and we need outsiders' perspectives. Flame Throwing is a great tool to test our idea. Flame Throwing corrects groupthink before it happens and bypasses most people's anxiety about receiving criticism. Flame Throwing provides an important opportunity to turn extreme negative feedback into constructive input in a fun way; it ritualizes the act of soliciting feedback, creates space for it and allows for actively ending criticism. Think of Flame Throwing as burning your concept down so you can lift it up to a new (high) level.

The mechanic of Flame Throwing comes from scriptwriting. Young writers are told to always bring a notebook when they get feedback on a story. Then, right after receiving a comment that triggers a defense response, the writer should break eye contact, lower his or her head and write the comment in the notebook. For starters it gives you a moment to regain your composure and counter the initial fight, flight or freeze reaction, but even more importantly when you're home the next day and you read it over in the safety of your own living room, you just might find that you agree with the feedback. Either way the feedback is not lost in the rush of blood that your animal brain is causing. So, drop your head, break eye contact and write it down!

How is Flame Throwing done? First, select outsiders as flamethrowers to pitch your concept to. Ask them to listen initially. Then, turn your back toward the flamethrowers and let them tear your concept apart. You're not allowed to defend your idea. Instead, sit back and listen. Take notes to capture feedback. Then, with your team, review all that feedback and see if you can improve your concept accordingly.

Fight, flight or freeze

The problem with listening to feedback is that it triggers a threat response. The older parts of our brain – the limbic system or mammalian brain – are usually the ones that are activated when we perceive something to be a threat. The possible responses have been categorized into three basic choices: fight, flight or freeze. It is a very physical phenomenon. It's instinctive, in that it happens without cognitive thought. The body prepares for the fight, flight or freeze choice by releasing extra hormones such as adrenaline and noradrenaline, increasing heart rates and blood pressure, dilating

(continued)

(continued)

pupils and slowing down other processes such as digestion. Just like an animal, we are physically ready to respond to danger.

Given that it is the animal part of us that is responding, think of the fight reaction as that of a cat that hisses and makes itself big with its hair on end and its back arched. The flight response is like the zebra running from a lion. The freeze response is that of the possum, famous for pretending to be dead when in danger.

Luckily, most of us are human enough when receiving feedback that we undergo verbal versions of these reactions: fighting with words, fleeing by agreeing to everything that is said, and freezing by shutting down and going out of contact.

Why does our mammal brain think it is necessary to get ready for such radical action? It is hard to argue with a zebra getting all worked up and running from a lion, but here we are just talking about feedback on an entrepreneurial idea. Why do we still think it is a matter of life and death?

According to clinical psychiatrist Elaine Aron, it has to do with the living conditions of our very distant ancestors (Aron, 1996). In the period when our brain was formed around 100,000 years ago, most of our ancestors lived in small tribes. Being rejected by your tribe meant certain death, and it was probably considered to be a fate worse than death. Our brains are thus still highly attuned to signs of social rejection and easily consider any signal of rejection to be a threat. Health entre-preneurship requires being aware of one's own responses to perceived threats and having the ability to consciously choose behavior that will disarm these responses.

Each response has a physical cue that can help you recognize it as soon as it happens. The fight response makes you want eye contact: you want to stare at the other. You sit or stand up straight and you feel lots of energy. The flight response is characterized by rapid and high breathing, lots of smiling and use of qualifiers such as "maybe" or "a little." In the freeze response, you feel as though you have lost contact with your own body. You might feel dizziness, your eyes focus on one point and you seek out activities you can do on automatic pilot.

Health entrepreneurship requires the ability to recognize and understand these reactions in others and especially in oneself as a leader. You will not be able to prevent fight-flight-freeze responses completely. The best thing to do is to have strategies ready for receiving feedback that compensate for these threat responses so that you can hear the feedback and learn from it. Let's look at two effective strategies and the tools to put these into practice in your health entrepreneurship journey.

Practical example

Our nutritionist asked some parents in the neighborhood to provide feedback on her farmers' market concept. First, she presented her idea, and then she let the people respond while she faces her back to them. This helped her not to defend her idea and to focus on learning from the feedback.

Call to action

You have 30 minutes to work with your team and any outsiders you deem appropriate to get feedback on your idea through the exercise of Flame Throwing.

Chapter 5

Prototyping

This chapter introduces the third phase of the Innovation Flow, Prototyping. Using the idea you identified in the Visioning phase, you need to get as much learning, input and feedback as fast as possible. Prototyping is about identifying what works and what doesn't work, moving the idea forward by creating different versions of it. This chapter guides your entrepreneurial journey as you:

- create quick and dirty representations of your idea;
- work with your hands to evolve your concept;
- go out into the world to interact with users and seek their reactions to your idea;
- get feedback, questions and new ideas from your users.

At the end of this Prototyping chapter, you will understand the concept of Prototyping, you will have explored the required mind-sets and you will have worked on your challenge with tools from the Prototyping tool kit (Hilberts, B2018). You will conclude this chapter with a further developed idea that you will take forward in the next step of your entrepreneurial journey: Scaling.

Introduction to Prototyping

It is extremely difficult to develop thoughtful solutions to complex health care challenges, never mind do so perfectly and get it right the first time. Hence Prototyping (Hilberts et al., 2014). Prototyping is quickly fabricating the envisioned solution, then iterating the solution multiple times. The cost of fabrication should be low, and your process of fabrication and testing should be rapid. Think tape, glue, cardboard, etc. Unlike most aspects of health care, we're not talking fancy or expensive. Just the opposite works best for Prototyping.

Prototyping has three important advantages. First, Prototyping makes the concept tangible. One can use all senses to design the proposed concept. Second, Prototyping is like thinking with your hands: it forces consistency and completeness, and by bringing your concept to life, you will encounter new questions, challenges and ideas that further shape your concept. Last, Prototyping triggers concrete and pointed feedback from users and experts. Especially if Prototyping is done in a fast and low-cost way, one can undertake multiple iterations and parallel experiments. Used this way, rapid Prototyping becomes a discovery tool of experiment, learning and improvement.

A "great" idea is thus the result of a long journey of bad ideas that triggers yet another iteration of a concept. Successful entrepreneurial ideas typically pivot (fundamentally changing your concept) at least three times. The saying is "success is going from failure to failure while never losing enthusiasm" (Powers, 1958). Failure is something to be celebrated in Prototyping, so long as the learnings from failure are captured and the prototype is improved as a result.

Initially, prototypes are unpolished, created from scrap materials at low costs. Toward the end of the process, prototypes evolve to become increasingly sophisticated. Prototypes become well-designed pilots for validating and falsifying critical assumptions that underpin the concept. Prototyping ends with confidence that the users will want the proposed solution and that you will generate a meaningful return.

During the Prototyping phase, the goal is to gather feedback with the aim of improving the concept and not validating it yet. Iterative trial, feedback and adaptation is key to this phase.

Receiving feedback

The role of feedback in entrepreneurship is well established: we need to know how we are performing, both in terms of content and in how we lead our team. Health entrepreneurs constantly seek and integrate feedback. There is an art to giving feedback. What about *receiving* feedback? Can health entrepreneurship mean not listening to feedback from time to time? How could you receive feedback in such a way that you benefit from it and don't feel cut down by it?

As a health entrepreneur changing the way that health care is delivered, you should probably worry if you are *not* being criticized. Health

(continued)

(continued)

entrepreneurship means getting things done, and for that you need to be out there in the arena, to be visible and to know that there will always be people at the sideline who will find something to say about you. Make your brain enjoy the fact that you are receiving feedback. You are in the arena and are getting noticed. Allow that fact by itself to strengthen your entrepreneurial drive.

Of course, there is more to it. Just being emboldened by this thought and happily ignoring feedback that comes your way is not the answer. Feedback can enhance your concept, help you gain insights into how to move forward, and help you become aware of parts of your concept that don't work yet.

It's all about being as playful as you can, being quick and dirty and cheap, show but don't tell, take on as much learning and feedback as you can and keep refining your idea. LinkedIn founder Reid Hoffman is famous for saying: "if you're not embarrassed by the first version of your product, you've launched too late" (Saint, 2009). We know these recommendations are countercultural to health care delivery. Let's be clear: SAFETY FIRST. We're not saying that you should be careless when health and lives are at stake or that you should ignore procedures and good practices. At the same time, there are many situations where you can safely try something new or let users experience a safe version of your concept. Safety is not an excuse for not Prototyping, it's a boundary condition.

Pull in users and experts as early as you can and as often as you can. Try not to defend your concept; rather, listen. Cherish feedback that you get as a gift – the feedback will help make your entrepreneurial ideas better. Celebrate failures, because really, they're just discoveries about ways to improve your concept. Continue to fail and experiment until you get to the big idea you're after.

Prototyping entails building a simple physical representation of the idea for feedback and improvement. A working product, or prototype, no matter how ugly or clunky – otherwise you are working only with assumptions. Avoid a prototype that is too polished. Users may assume it's the final version. A key benefit of scale modelling is that it gets a user and/or expert to engage with the concept first-handedly to solicit direct feedback. Let users physically interact with your prototype. Invite them to try things in this "test drive." Let go of your prototypes physically and don't defend your prototype. Your job is to solicit feedback and leverage it to create an improved version again and again and again.

Prototyping is a crucial activity in entrepreneurship that is easily overlooked, underestimated or avoided:

- *Easily overlooked:* once an entrepreneur has a promising new idea, the temptation is to go for a quick launch without wasting any more time. But time spent on Prototyping is a strategic investment since your entrepreneurial idea has improved odds for success. Buyers will have been consulted and their feedback incorporated – you know they want it since they have co-created it.

- *Easily underestimated*: Prototyping may look child-ish, especially in the early stages when the toys and fun could be misconstrued as a playful activity without business benefits. Early-stage Prototyping will, however, ensure that potential flaws are dis-covered early on, when they are not yet costly to repair. Upon market introduction, it will be too late to repair them cheaply.

- *Easily avoided*: we want to avoid the pain or loss of face often associated with failure – and we will fail a lot during Prototyping. Reframing failure as a starting point to learn and improve from, rather than a result to be ashamed of, will go a long way to overcoming the natural hesitation many of us feel toward failure.

Prototyping is a serious job. It has serious benefits in the serious quest for entrepreneurial breakthroughs. The playful spirit that goes along with Prototyping is functional in that it creates safety to fail, encour-ages creativity and fuels the energy needed to keep on making iterations. The fact that even the most senior executives also have a whale of a time during Prototyping is a pleasant side effect. Avoid pitfalls, and just go for it. Build! Break! Try! Play! Dare! And let us know what works for you.

Prototyping is not market research

Unmet user needs are considered the holy grail of prod-uct and service innovation: a mystical, sacred entity with unlimited value and powers for those that know how to tap into it. With present day digitalization and social media, it is easier to connect to users everywhere through online surveys, platforms and data mining technology. Moving from a mass-producing economy to one based on individually tailored products suggests that the gap between user needs and producer response is closely aligned. Yet the mystique surrounding unmet user needs remains: the recent study by Philippe Duverger shows that the gap between users and product developers continues to exist (Duverger, 2012). The study reiterates the need to find effective ways to include users in product and service creation to secure future innovation, and warns that if companies fail to do so, business will suffer.

Indeed, the need to include users (i.e. patients or others involved in the health system like parents, visitors or employees) in product and business design is clear, yet we continue to argue that people often do not know what they really want, really need or are really missing. As the first car manufacturer Henry Ford once said, "if I'd asked people what they wanted, they would have said a faster horse." The lesson here isn't to ask customers what they want, for they may not know. It's about coming up with concepts that might solve their problems and then showing them these concepts and getting their response. That means developing what *The Lean Startup* author Eric Ries calls a minimum viable product, testing different versions and gathering feedback (Ries, 2011).

Prototyping support

There is a rich variety of powerful, low-cost opportunities for rapid Prototyping. These are different in their resolution or in how similar they are to the end product. Remember to Prototype as low resolution and as cheap as possible in the beginning and work your way up to more realistic prototypes over time.

Toys

Children's toys are effective tools for rapid Prototyping – especially in the early stages of the process. These range from LEGO and Play-Doh (Scale Model Prototypes), to crayons (Storyboard Prototypes) and costumes (Role-Play Prototypes). littleBits and Cubelets are a bit more advanced, and good to use when simple electronic or robotic functions are desired.

You will need to step over the hesitation to use simple materials or toys on health care concepts that are serious and may entail life or death scenarios. We have had to overcome our own hesitations to find that that even very senior executives at large corporations will do this successfully and with a lot of verve. They did not look like they thought it was a waste of their precious time. Release your inner entrepreneur: it knows what it means to be creative and the joy of entrepreneurship.

3-D printing

3-D printing, FabLabs, etc. nowadays cost as little as office equipment and are simple enough to be used directly by entrepreneurship building its own prototypes instead of having to resort to specialists. You can easily outsource 3-D printing to a designer and printer with a simple online search for options.

Virtual reality

3-D modelling, drawing tools (e.g. SketchUp), or online games (e.g. SimCity) can model and simulate an idea on a laptop. These tools are typically available at low cost, with fast turnaround time. More advanced system dynamics computer simulations are very powerful and sufficiently unstructured to allow for surprise learning. SimCity is a great tool to prototype with for ideas around cities, mobility and communities.

Online feedback

Online surveys and online panels are simple to create and show quick results. SurveyMonkey is a useful free resource to design a simple survey to enlist people to provide online feedback. Quantitative feedback can be useful in rating different versions of a prototype or of a prototype feature. One needs to step over the ambition of proper market research; entrepreneurship at this phase means that you look for insights, not statistical validation. The survey should include fields for qualitative feedback.

The Prototyping mind-sets

Prototyping means adopting several mind-sets. Some of these mind-sets go against deeply ingrained ways of working and behaving in health care, so we have to keep reminding ourselves of them.

Celebrate failure

We usually resist failure – we are hardwired to avoid it, especially in health care where people's lives are at stake. But failure should be actively pursued in Prototyping. If the prototype runs smoothly, nothing new will be learned, yet Prototyping is all about learning. Failures are to be expected and entrepreneurship seeks failure. The key is to get feedback about what went wrong, learn from the situation and get it right on a future try. In short, keys to failure entail:

- fail often;
- fail forward;
- learn from failure to move forward with an improved version;
- fail as early as possible;
- fail as cheaply as possible.

Consider the Post-its that we have been using so much in the Visioning phase. The Post-it came about by an engineer at 3M who tried to invent very strong glue. He obviously failed miserably. But rather than hiding his failure and sweeping his mistake under the carpet, he celebrated it. He shared his mistakes with his colleagues and one of them – a singer in a choir – saw benefits. This colleague mentioned a problem of losing his hymn notes in his church choir book. He suggested to use the glue on the backs of paper so that they could be stuck and removed without leaving residue, which was the start of how Post-it notes came to be.

Think with your hands

Building a concrete and tangible prototype taps a different source of creativity. When the creator moves his energy from his head to his hands, the idea often improves. Same with health care: when the clinician moves her energy from her head to her hands, the patient (ideally) improves. When done in a creative team, this is the point at which team members get aligned around the idea. Building the prototype surfaces potential misunderstandings, different interpretations or assumptions, and then resolves them. By thinking with your hands, your inner entrepreneur is unlocked. This entrepreneur loves to create new things and is not hindered by the inner critic who wonders how other people might react to it. Play and fun are positive forces of health care entrepreneurship.

Bias toward action

There is an inherent sense of urgency in health care because there is no time to lose when human life is on the line. Entrepreneurship must avoid paralysis through analysis. Stop talking about it and do it, build it! One of the big insights from data about Prototyping contests is that teams that start building immediately end up with better results than teams that analyze and plan before they start building (van Dijk et al., 2015). The mere act of moving out of their brain and into their hands makes all the difference. When you build a prototype, you release creativity and rally the team around the idea.

Iterate

The magic and power of Prototyping comes out in iterations: going over the process again and again. This goes against our desire to develop finished products, which are right the first time around. Once we shift our mind-set to the idea of multiple iterations, playfulness and experimentation can begin. We know that whatever we add or adapt will be short-lived, until the next iteration. A product with many iterations will always be superior to a product that is painstakingly designed to be as finished as possible.

Rough around the edges

A prototype is never really finished – it gets replaced in the next iteration. It doesn't need to be polished, to be complete or to look good. A prototype is eternally a work-in-progress. It should look unfinished, as if it has just been cobbled together with whatever was at hand. Learn to love the rough aspect of prototypes. They belong in the background, not on the front lines of health care delivery.

Entrepreneurship in action: SickKids

The Hospital for Sick Children in Toronto treats children from cancer. The challenge they faced was to get children to fill out detailed pain journals every day. In their Sensing, the team identified that the treatment often makes the children feel too feeble, tired or disheartened to actually write these reports. This low compliance is a problem since it leads to suboptimal treatment – as understanding and managing pain levels increases patient well-being, costs efficiency and treatment efficacy. They reframed their problem to look not for incentives to drive compliance but for intrinsic motivation to drive engagement.

In their Visioning process, the team generated many ideas including gamifying the experience, using characters that kids can relate to and that take their minds off their illness and creating exclusive content that only they could access. In Prototyping their idea, they tested multiple themes and a platform to deliver content and track data. These were tested in an analogue way, with a mock-up of a diary. The feedback was most positive about a detective theme. The theme feedback and platform feedback helped to settle on a mobile app called Pain Squad, in which a "special police force" dedicated to ridding the world of pain invites them to file a report twice a day. The app includes game mechanics like promotions and awards. The story is brought to life by famous actors from top-rated police dramas who engage the kids in activities and encourage them for a job well done. The story is not just engaging, it provides a purpose and transforms the mind-set of the kids into pain fighters rather than just information reporters. The results of this project were significantly higher compliance rates in filling out the pain reports which in turn led to better pain treatment and better care outcomes.

Challenge: start Prototyping

Now it's time to train that bias toward action on the topic you and your team have been working on. The rest of this chapter takes you through several Prototyping tools that help you create prototypes, gather feedback and learn more.

Tool 18: Storyboarding

In Storyboarding, we sketch the user experience for feedback and improvement. We use Storyboarding when we want to get away from words, leave room for interpretation and when we want fast feedback.

Don't worry if you feel you cannot draw. Most people are not afull-time artists; that's not the point. All of us have the power to create stick drawings and sketch something that others can understand. Remember that if you're not embarrassed you've spent too much time. Now let's craft a narrative of how the user will experience the concept. Select –four to six evocative "moments of truth" in this narrative to sketch, like a comic book. Start with the first moment, then sketch the last moment and then fill out the rest of the journey.

Practical example

For the farmers' market in school idea, a team member of the nutritionist quickly sketched what the user experience looked like.

This not only allowed the team to explain the concept to others and to get their feedback, it also made

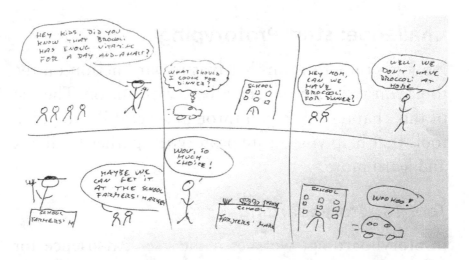

FIGURE 5.1 Storyboard example

clear to the team that it wasn't just about the convenience of buying groceries while picking up your kids, there was also the opportunity to have the farmers partake in the educational process.

Call to action

Take 30 minutes with your team to create a storyboard. Remember it needs to be rough around the edges and remember that this is thinking with your hands: so your concept can still evolve while making the storyboard.

Tool 19: Scale Modelling

Scale Modelling allows you to work with your hands. Use this tool when you need a tangible manifestation of your concept to make it easier to show what you're envisioning and receive direct feedback.

Be ready to play. Build a quick and dirty mash-up using whatever you've got around you. Avoid anything that's too polished, otherwise users may assume that it's the final version and they won't give enough feedback. We're talking playdough, foam, cardboard and glue. You can even use yourself and your team to create a role-play that people can experience. Seriously, this is a mock-up. Create versions of your idea to parallel test options within the concept that remain undecided.

Practical example

For the farmers' market in school idea, the nutritionist built a LEGOmodel of a school cafeteria with the farmers' market and the routing for the children vis-à-vis the rest of the cafeteria.

Call to action

Take 30 minutes with your team to build your first scale model. Remember it needs to be rough around the edges and remember that this is thinking with your hands: so your concept can still evolve while making the storyboard.

Tool 20: User Prototype Test

Let's assume we've got our prototype. Now we need to test it to see if the prototype works, not just for us, but for others too. If the prototype doesn't work, we want to fail quickly and cheaply. Testing the prototype with users helps determine if you're building the right "it" before you build it right. This process enables both users and experts to interact with the prototype and provide measurable feedback.

Use a low-resolution mock-up, preferably two to three different versions which highlight different features. Invite users for a "test drive," and then create a safe space where they feel comfortable giving honest, critical feedback. Encourage users to actively engage with your prototype and interact with them where possible while using the prototype. Observe how users engage with the prototype and what they struggle with. Try not to interfere too much. Solicit feedback and try and capture it in a feedback grid with four categories: what users like, what users don't like, the questions the prototype raises and the new ideas it evokes. If you don't get a lot of feedback from your user, you can use these categories to formulate questions: "What do you like about this concept?", "What do you miss about this concept?", "What questions do you have?" and

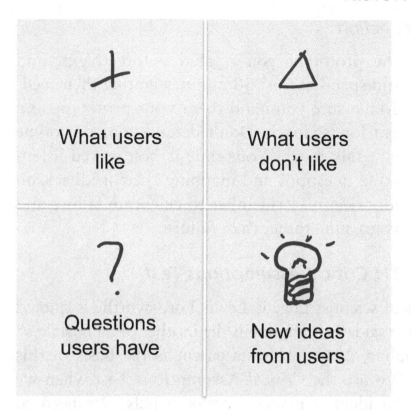

FIGURE 5.2 Feedback grid

"What ideas do you have to make it better?" Leverage the feedback into an improved version. Iterate for continuous improvement.

Practical example

Using our concept of a farmers' market in a school, one of the prototypes that our nutritionist made was a scale model. She invited teachers, children and parents and put the farmers' market in the middle while asking them about how it would work. She documented their feedback without defending our model and iterated the concept further with her team.

Call to action

Take the prototype you created before. Next, find users and spend at least 30 minutes getting their feedback. Make sure you hand them your prototype and ask them for feedback. Don't defend your prototype and don't talk much. Your time is best served listening, asking questions and mapping their feedback on the feedback grid. Remember to celebrate failure and see it as learning rather than failure.

Tool 21: Critical Assumptions Test

Political scientist Eugene Lewis Fordsworthe is quoted to have said: "assumption is the mother of all mistakes" (Prabahar, 2011). This statement is the basis of this tool. We use the Critical Assumptions Test when we want to identify make-or-break beliefs. We need to reassure other people's concerns about the idea and be satisfied about the feasibility of our concept.

So the great things about the Critical Assumptions Test is that it brings to the surface and tests the have-to-believe assumptions that were made during the Visioning process. The Critical Assumptions Test reduces the risks of reactive, uncertain and edgy concepts by confirmation of validity or plausibility around these assumptions. And it assures you that you have fixed the weak spots and identified flaws before making substantial investments and entering the market.

Here's how you do your Critical Assumptions Test. Identify and select the key make-or-break assumptions underpinning your concept, and ask yourself the question, "What do we have to believe for this concept to become successful?" Answers typically revolve around

Desirability (do users really want this product or service?), Viability (will we be able to deliver it in a way where costs and benefits make sense?) and Feasibility (is it possible from technological, legal, process and other perspectives?). When you have identified your make-or-break assumptions, create a test to find proof that validates or falsifies each of the assumptions. Testing could be many things, from internet research to expert interviews to staging a quick and dirty market test. Alternatively, find examples from different situations to demonstrate the plausibility. Fix problems now, before a critical assumption turns out to be invalid or not plausible. Go back to the Visioning process if you need to.

Practical example

Our nutritionist and her team set out a long-list of assumptions and prioritized the assumption that children would eat more fruit and vegetables if there was a farmers' market. To test this assumption they designed an experiment: they would ask school staff to measure average fruit and vegetable consumption in one local school for a week and they would enlist a local farmer to create a farmers' market the next week and measure the difference.

Call to action

Gather your team, brainstorm assumptions that you have made in the categories desirability, viability and feasibility and prioritize them. Now design experiments to validate or falsify the prioritized assumptions. Remember the bias toward action: design your test in a way that you can execute it fast.

Chapter 6

Scaling

We're in the last phase of the Innovation Flow: Scaling. This means you've identified what your users need in Sensing, you've generated a concept that serves that need in Visioning and you've improved that concept through feedback in Prototyping. Now you're ready to enrich your concept with ways to make it scale, spread or go viral. Scaling is all about coming up with small, smart moves that generate outsized results. This chapter guides your next step on the entrepreneurial journey as you:

- enrich your concept with small smart moves to maximize impact;
- implement simple tactics that influence the system and create emerging patterns;
- leverage network effects to improve the outcomes for your concept;
- harness the energy that is inherent in the system to accelerate your success.

At the end of this Scaling chapter, you will understand the concept of Scaling, you will have explored the required mind-sets and you will have worked on your challenge with tools from the Scaling tool kit (Hilberts, 2018). You will conclude this chapter with a concept that can scale and is ready for the next step: Creating Action.

Introduction to Scaling

When you have a new entrepreneurial concept, you want it to be successful. You want many people and organizations to buy the product, use the service or adopt your new approach. Scaling is the process of designing smart elements into your product or service so that they scale better.

We have divided this topic into three main areas: Emergence, Networks and Waves. Emergence refers to the phenomenon of patterns becoming apparent in complex systems of interacting agents. Entrepreneurship can look to make use of emergent collective behavior by designing openness into a system and designing rules for interaction, which allow successful behavior to surface and spread. Networks refer to the properties of networks, the structures and technology supporting networks and the social conditioning that exists with network members to scale their innovations. Waves are a naturally occurring phenomenon in complex systems. It is one thing for entrepreneurs to be prepared to watch for waves and catch them when they appear. It is another thing altogether to create, nurture and sustain waves that are steered in the direction of your entrepreneurial vision.

The health care market is composed of a system of connected users. Smartly designed interventions can spread rapidly and might trigger a big impact. Entrepreneurial concepts designed to incorporate infectious effects can spread like the flu. Concepts that are timed to launch and coincide with external momentum can ride this wave to success. Well-designed Scaling tactics could mean that the outcome goes beyond the concept conceived to spark a self-propelling movement around it, which drastically reduces the effort and costs to sustain the success.

This chapter will lean heavily on examples outside the health care industry. As we said in Chapter 2, do not be put off by these entrepreneurial ideas from other industries if they seem out of line with your health care experience. Health entrepreneurship will benefit from exposure to entrepreneurial thinking that is interdisciplinary, thinking that has worked well in other industries and can be applied in the ripe-for-disruption health care industry.

The rules of emergence (van Asseldonk et al., 2014)

Understanding collective behavior is becoming more important for health entrepreneurship as there are increasing levels of complexity in the health care system. This is fueled by the ever-increasing connectivity between parts of the system and the growth of available big data to inform feedback loops. In complex systems, top-down control is not an effective answer. It is much more effective to understand the rules that seem to govern the system. Systems always have a set of behavioral rules, or the interactions in the system will be chaos. Such behavioral rules guide the capacity for self-organizing.

There are some famous biological examples of system rules. Ants in colonies are apparently effectively working together without central command and control to feed the population. Computer simulations have demonstrated that such collaborative colony behavior occurs by the application of three simple rules: (1) move randomly, (2) if you pick up a scent from another ant follow that upstream (ants leave a scent trail from the food source to the nest) and (3) if you find another ant struggling with a task, help him. It is unknown whether this is really what's going on in the ant's brain, but it does produce striking patterns of behavior. Similarly, a few simple rules seem to cause birds to fly in a flock, even when they don't know about flocks.

An illustration outside the animal kingdom is the working of roundabouts. During the best part of the 20th century, mainland Europe established the "give way to the right" and the "keep on the right side" laws combined with a system rule where cars had *priority when wanting to get on* the roundabout, because cars driving on the roundabout had to give way to cars entering the roundabout from their right. In the UK, however, a different system rule emerged. The "give way to the right" and "keep on the left side" laws combined to a system rule where you had *priority when you are already on* the roundabout. This time the cars on the roundabout came from the right, they had priority over those wanting to get on and thus could clear the roundabout quickly. The differences in efficiency and safety were substantial, basically the system rule created efficient self-organizing traffic flows within a wide range of conditions. It took a long time to understand the benefits of changing the system rules to make it work in the rest of Europe. By using signage to clarify the priority on mainland roundabouts from "priority when wanting to get on" to "priority when already on," the desired system outcome of fluid traffic flow with fewer accidents emerged. The impact is huge, as many crossings that used to be controlled by traffic lights are now equipped with roundabouts with "priority when already on" rules. You can take away the expensive top-down control mechanisms of traffic lights because the self-organizing system with the right rules works better.

The structure of networks (Turrell et al., 2014)

Human behavior is strongly affected and shaped by the way people are connected together. Our life is full of networks. There are physical networks, as the neural network of brains, the electrical power grid, the pager network in a hospital and the World Wide Web. There are activity networks, national hospital networks and global trade networks. And there are social networks, which are defined by all different types of communities to which people can belong: friendship networks, professional networks, etc. It is this latter category of networks that is most relevant for Scaling: both the physical version and the online version of social networks.

Entrepreneurship leverages social networks for Scaling. Possibly the most important aspect of networks when thinking of Scaling is diffusion, e.g. the spreading of new products, services and entrepreneurial ideas, but also of information and of social behaviors. Entrepreneurship aims to spread new ideas rapidly through a web of connected nodes and overlapping networks. To do so successfully, it is important to understand the structure of a social network you may be targeting to leverage.

Each network consists of nodes and links that connect the nodes. In social networks, the nodes are people, the links are conversations through communication channels, such as email messages, telephone calls or pager requests. Nodes with many connections are "hubs" and thus can serve as "bridges" to nodes with lower connectivity. When entrepreneurs want to use networks for diffusion of messages or new ideas, it works better in networks that have larger variance in connectivity, which means that some nodes have few links and others have many links. The intuition is that even a limited number of nodes with many links allows the transmission of the diffusion, working as "bridges" between regions of nodes with lower connectivity. When a social network has centrally located clusters, messages or ideas also spread easier.

The energy of waves (Turrell et al., 2014)

Brian Arthur, one of the pioneers of positive feedback economics, has a favorite story. Born in Hawaii and a skilled surfer, Arthur explains that the key to good surfing is the ability to spot an adequate wave as it forms. That gives you time to reach the right place to catch the wave. The capability of riding the wave is only half of what is needed; spotting it in the first place is essential.

The existence of waves is visible in everyday life. Whether it is in "Trending Topics" on Twitter or preseason fashion trends, new elements suddenly surface and grow into system-wide expressions and manifestations, or new trends in music and entertainment. If many people go and see a movie, we deem it to be interesting, even if we were initially hesitant to go. In case of fire we all run to the same fire exit.

In many cases the causes of such waves are very difficult to track. The existence of such waves is a direct expression of the effect of interaction and positive feedback, where small causes can lead to system-wide consequences. As in wave surfing, entrepreneurship requires the skill to detect such emerging waves in time to get on top of them.

In addition, if entrepreneurship understands the underlying forces and creates a small but determining change in the working of the system, it may provide a very powerful tool in using the wave energy. Companies have done so successfully in the past. Benetton ("United Colors of Benetton") sensed the growing trend of individualism in clothing. To accommodate this from the classical setup of the manufacturing process (first coloring the garment and then knitting it into the final product) was not economical. It required a level of prediction and planning that was no longer compatible with the heterogeneous and unpredictable nature of the markets they wanted to serve. They showed entrepreneurship by developing the technology to reverse these two manufacturing steps, enabling them to color the sweaters driven by consumer choice in the outlets, after production and immediately before delivery.

When the Impact Hub was started in London in 2005, it exhibited entrepreneurship by riding a dual wave of social entrepreneurship and the trend toward more self-employed or small startup professionals. Seven years later, there is a network of more than 25 hubs across five continents, providing a place where entrepreneurs can go to work, learn and network. Their telltale slogan is "Where change goes to work." Spaces are designed to provide a creative environment, as well as a professional environment. Membership is customized from people who work there full time, to those who solely attend the events. Users have access to Impact Hub locations across the world.

These Scaling frames offer health care entrepreneurs tactics to favorably influence the emergence of successful outcomes. They do so by leveraging the notion that a lot of pent-up energy is available in current health care systems that will carry your concept when released. Skillful health care entrepreneurs aim to spot, catch and ride a big wave, and will try to create a movement with its own rhythm, building toward its own nexus to make it unavoidable for people to join. As the right waves fundamentally boost new ideas or products, efforts to build an inevitable climax can have an outsized impact.

Though it is no guarantee for success, consciously designing for scale will give health entrepreneurs a better position to benefit from Scaling opportunities than by depending on chance.

The Scaling mind-sets

Scaling is both an opportunistic and a strategic phase; you need to keep an open mind to opportunities, listen well to what's going on in the system around, be strategic about leveraging these insights and you can co-create interventions with others. In Scaling, we therefore see two mind-sets come back that we have seen before in Sensing and Visioning.

Postpone judgment

The health care system is riddled with pressure: pressure to cut budgets, time pressure to fit in more patients and time pressure to cure as fast as possible. This leads to the need to quickly judge the facts of a situation, recognize patterns and define a solution or treatment. During Sensing, you need the exact opposite. Only when you release your agenda and remain completely open to all possibilities, will you be truly receptive to new learning. This is exceptionally hard to do for people who work in result-oriented, time-pressured environments – i.e. health care. Yet health entrepreneurship means knowing that the moment you believe you know the answer or form a judgment, you will be obstructing the view of the unexpected, and risk missing out on serendipitous encounters.

Truly listening without judging is not an easy task. It helps to force yourself to listen for what you do not want to hear. For instance, if a team is excited about a new opportunity space, it might be tempted to close its ears to those saying, "we tried that already in the past and it failed." However, if you force yourself to listen, you have an interesting Sensing opportunity to delve into experience and draw learning from it. The other way around, the fact that you didn't succeed in solving a certain situation before does not mean you can't find a different way to solve it today.

Yes and . . .

The divergent part of Visioning is primarily a social process. You cannot really brainstorm alone and often one person just has half an idea that only becomes good if it's combined with another person's idea. To make this collaboration successful, it's key to not challenge or dismiss ideas of others. Rather encourage people by acknowledging all ideas (even the craziest) and by building on them. In other words: always say "Yes and . . ." rather than "Yes but . . ."

Entrepreneurship in action: the Aravind Eye Hospitals and Clinics

As we learned in reading the previous chapters, the Aravind Eye Hospitals and Clinics in India revolutionized the entire system of providing eye surgeries with astonishing results both in financial terms and in terms of health outcomes. The Aravind Eye Hospitals and Clinics in India have been helping the blind population with access to high-quality care at affordable rates. Part of their success stemmed from the eye-care camps that were held several thousand times each year as discussed in the Sensing chapter. Taking from this position of impact, the clinic wanted to better understand how to scale. As the clinic investigated how much of an impact they were having, they realized they were only hitting 7% of the population. Without a doubt the work they were doing was not only impressive but it was also impactful. But to have more impact meant Scaling their operations.

The success of the clinic stemmed from smart decisions that were spread rapidly and accelerated adoption through the spread of information across communities. And while the clinic was providing thousands of community eye-care camps each year to create a large scale impact and support the community needs they needed to make strategic decisions and leverage the community social dynamics. The success that they had built created a showcase to trigger further growth. Something different needed to happen.

Vision centers were opened throughout surrounding communities. These are truly paperless offices focused on completely using electronic medical records. Telemedicine technology was also deployed. The teleconference using video occurred between patients in the vision center and the medical officers in the base hospital. A simple digital camera was turned into an eye examination camera. Within the first year of appointment there was a 40% penetration into the market that was served, which is approximately 50,000 people. The second year it grew to 75% of market penetration. The scale was to focus on reaching every person who needed care. The leveraging of technology ensured that most individuals did not need to come to the base hospital. For three consults they paid about Rs.20, which in today's equivalence is less than US$.50, the pricing factored in what they would save in bus fare needed to go to the base hospital. To provide this high tech medical access in rural areas, it was necessary to design a van equipped with these services to allowgreater access. The report of the findings is sent back to the patient while they are still waiting after their consultation and next steps are provided. This has been an effective way to bridge the technology competence. Growth was focused on reaching the unreachable and therefore significantly growing the market. Additionally, with the limited resources of the ophthalmologists, they have set up the operations in such a way thatwhen one surgery is complete the second patient is prepped and ready immediately behind the ophthalmologist's current patient. A microscope is flipped over and the ophthalmologist is ready to go with the next patient. Minor details are accounted for, such as ensuring that the gap between the patients is just right. This has allowed the productivity of of the surgeons to quadruple.

Thinking upstream, an additional 300 individuals are recruited from the local communities each year and trained to act as the backbone of the organization. Their support role is to administer all of the skill-based routine tasks. They focus on doing one thing at a time and focus on doing it extremely well. This results in a very high productivity achieved at a high quality and low cost. The productivity of this clinic not only outshined that of any other in India but of the surrounding countries as well. Complication rates are also significantly less than those that have been reported in the United Kingdom.

The success of Scaling also rests on having a strong financial foundation. The clinic was able to achieve their scale in their success by finding a way to make it affordable and most importantly sustainable for their new markets. This included offering many of their services for free for those who could not afford the services and those who paid local market rates. This philosophy stemmed from having a value system built around giving away what you have as a surplus. What this equated to over time is that expenses have increased and so have the revenues, however the revenues have increased at a higher rate than the expenses providing for a healthy margin.

Challenge: start designing for Scale

In the previous chapter, you received feedback on your prototypes and were able to refine your concept. Now is the time to bake in some of the Scaling mechanics that will allow your concept to get traction fast. The rest of this chapter takes you through several practical tools to do so.

Tool 22: Emergence Scaling Frames

We have selected four Emergence Scaling Frames. They form examples of how emergence takes place and how others have used emergence to their advantage. These examples are not from the health care industry, but nonetheless, they can form inspiration for your project. Each Scaling frame consists of a description, an example and a set of trigger questions to guide your thinking.

Balance control

Define the core features that you believe you must provide and control yourself, while enabling configuration and personalization for the other areas of your offering. Enlarge your potential market by allowing adaptation and configuration of product features – either by the users or by other players in the product's or service's ecosystem. Your offering can support a wide variety of user experiences and stir feelings of co-ownership and actions toward shared success.

Example:

- Salesforce.com, ranked the most innovative company in the US by Forbes in 2013, is an enterprise software company based in San Francisco. It has over 100,000 different paying customers. Salesforce.com offers its clients an increasing selection of software solutions.
- The only way the company can efficiently meet such a large variety of customer needs and carry on growing, is to allow for high levels of configuration for all of its products.
- Many software firms follow this route, and by providing SDKs (software development kits) they enable third parties to design their own products, features and application combinations whilst complying with a core set of requirements from the software vendor.

Trigger questions:

- Which features and functionalities are so core to your offering that you never want to compromise on them?
- Which features and functionalities will you consciously make available for configuration and personalization by partners?
- How will you explicitly invite partners to (re-)configure the features that are open to them in their own style?

Balance control

Leverage data and analytics from a wide range of sources to uncover opportunities for Scaling. Use business intelligence tools to mine data for insights that may not be apparent or are obscured by too much noise in the data set. Success of this approach requires a diligent data collection and analysis mentality and capability, a sense of where to look for patterns and a willingness to recognize the results.

Example:

- McDonald's aggregated data from experimenting in three replica restaurants, leveraging sales data but also observations from volunteers acting as customers.
- By analyzing the aggregated data, McDonald's was able to assess the impact of new ideas, such as new menu items or a change in the location of the tills.

Trigger questions:

- How will you collect relevant data on the usage of your product?
- How can you tap into new sources of data to get a more complete picture of opportunities for Scaling?
- How will you develop intelligent analytical capabilities to make sense of this sea of data?

Design choices

Choice design nudges people toward the best option most of the time, with the least amount of effort and risk of disengaging. Design structured choices that steer your users toward those options that make it easier to scale, at the same time giving them the freedom to make choices in their own interest. For example, setting default options or labelling a package "most popular" on online order forms or tacitly encouraging people to continue with a service, such as small monthly subscription fees charged to a credit card.

(continued)

(continued)

Example:	Trigger questions:
• The city of Washington, DC intended to lower plastic bag consumption and therefore enacted a law forcing customers to pay five cents per plastic carrier bag. At the same time, stores reduced client demand by removing plastic bags from the checkout area, requiring customers to expressly ask for them in front of their fellow shoppers. This changed shoppers' default behavior to not using plastic bags.	• What is the user's end-to-end decision-making process and what are key choice points in this process?
	• What is the desired behavior at each choice point – and the undesired?
	• How can you make otherwise explicit choices become implicit – favoring the desired choice?
• Within the first six months, plastic bag consumption had fallen from 130 million bags to just 25 million, with 66% fewer bags found polluting the local river.	

Allow emergence

Allow new ideas to surface and evolve through exposure and use, and spread or disappear through often magical-seeming properties of the complex system of users. Deliberately provide space for experimentation and user choice. Allow users to highlight preferred concepts through feedback loops (e.g. encourage users to review and rate your concepts).

Example:

- Flickr emerged from community tools originally created for a massively multiplayer online game (MMOG) called "Game Neverending." Users could chat with each other using instant messaging windows and share digital images of objects in the game. This functionality was soon extended and rapidly users started to share photos.
- Eventually it became clear that the original vision of a game with an instant messaging environment was not what users valued and instead the need for photo sharing emerged. The team dropped the other features to focus on this functionality.
- According to co-founder, Caterina Fake: "Had we sat down and said, 'Let's start a photo application,' we would have failed, we would have done all this research and done all the wrong things."

Trigger questions:

- How will you install feedback mechanisms from users to highlight their preferences (and dislikes) of features and functionalities?
- How will you mentally prepare yourself for a pivot around an unplanned but emergent incarnation of your idea?

Practical example

For the farmers' market in school idea, the nutritionist read the Scaling frame called Balance Control and realized that rather than organizing a farmers' market in every single school, she could create a tool kit for schools to help them with organizing it themselves. This tool kit would consisted of best practices, contacts to find local farmers, predesigned display materials and posters and standard contract templates.

Call to action

Take 45 minutes with your team to go through each of the Scaling frames above and generate interventions to make your concept scale. Remember to postpone judgment and build on each other by saying yes and . . .

Tool 23: Networks Scaling Frames

We have selected four Scaling frames on networks. Each is an example of how you can design and leverage networks to make your concept scale and go viral. These examples are not from the health care industry, but nonetheless, they can form inspiration for your project. Each Scaling frame consists of a description, an example and a set of trigger questions to guide your thinking.

Jump across networks

Expand beyond the comfort zone of your own network and actively make connections and foster interactions with individuals with whom you are only remotely associated and who have moved through different careers, industries or disciplines. Network asks passed through these individuals can spread extremely quickly across different and additional geographic and industry boundaries than your own.

Example:

- The World Economic Forum created the Young Global Leader community and the Global Shaper community, both made up of "ultra-travelers."

Trigger questions:

- What other industries or geographies could be particularly relevant for your Scaling? Who do you know that can help you get there?

- The level of experience and diversity characterizing these communities makes them ideal places to connect with individuals to jump across networks and reach massive scale in a short amount of time.

- Who in your network could you reach out to for support in being introduced into new networks?

Infect with ideas

Learn from the spread of diseases and think about how your ideas and desired actions can be passed from one person to the next and from one to many. Think about your initiative as a virus, a disease that wants to spread, and craft your tactics so that they include factors to boost the likelihood of infection and the size of population that can be infected. Make contagion visible to everyone, so it becomes hard to ignore (e.g. "this message was sent from my iPad").

Example:

- Comic Relief is a British charity aiming to bring about positive and lasting change in the lives of poor and disadvantaged people. Its main fundraising event, Red Nose Day, is designed to spread like a virus.
- First run in 1988, Red Nose Day encourages people to buy and wear red noses, a very visible sign of inclusion that creates a certain peer pressure to join in. Schools often run red-nose-themed events, and a special catchy song has

Trigger questions:

- What is the action you ask users to undertake?
- What is a visible signal that people can display to signal that they are "infected"?
- How long/often do people need to be exposed to your message

(continued)

(continued)

shows all evening (parodies of recent popular shows, films and clips, events and specially filmed versions of comedy shows), presented by celebrity teams.	before they are ready to take the desired action?

Leverage network effects

Design your concept so that overall value of the network and the benefits to individuals increase with every new additional user in a nonlinear way. Initiatives that naturally incorporate connection and user interaction are likely to have network effects, such as the phone, the fax and social media. Positive user experiences are likely to generate further spread due to existing members bringing in new users, which in turn reinforces their positive perception of the service.

Example:

- The Android phone operating system, offered for free by Google, benefits from massive adoption and had achieved a 75% market share of smartphones by 2012. Google Play, the integrated app store, encourages more and more software developers onto the platform, as the core user base has been increasing at a rate of 1.5 million activations per day. At the same time, the availability of more apps makes these phones more interesting to customers, leading to additional users. Additional users make it more interesting for app

Trigger questions:

- What can you build into your offering so that it gets more valuable for existing users with each additional user that is added?
- How can you quickly get to a critical mass and reach a tipping point?
- What can you do to keep your users active and prevent passive connections ("lurking")?

developers to develop new versions for Android in addition to iPhone.

- In contrast, Nokia failed to grow its smartphone user base to the critical mass threshold, so that its attempts at app and music stores, originally branded Ovi, did not gain traction. In 2013, Nokia moved out of the mobile phone business by selling its operations to Microsoft.

Gamify

Use games, simulations, rewards and a sense of fun to offer an engaging platform for the user to learn, to process information, to connect to others or to make decisions. Engage with people on an emotional and playful level, even for more serious topics. People can become ever more hooked into your concept through "levels" or "points" that gradually increase the sophistication of use and move users up the proficiency curve.

Example:

- WASH United (WASH standing for Water, Sanitation and Hygiene) aims to end the global sanitation and hygiene crisis by making toilets and good hygiene "cool" and "exy."
- The World Toilet Cup is a real-world game of football where players have to kick the ball (or "poo ball"), penalty style, into toilet holes in a canvas.

Trigger questions:

- What games are your users already engaged in, how could you tie into these games?
- What are different game mechanics to incorporate, such as incentives (badges), stages (levels), etc.

(continued)

133

(continued)

- The Great WASH Yatra was an India-wide program in 2012 to boost awareness of the relevance of sanitation and hygiene. More than 160,000 people visited the carnival at its six stops. There were 20 different sanitation and hygiene programs. More than 152 schools were trained in good WASH behavior through the Yatra's WASH in Schools interventions.

- What is an advanced way of using your concept? Can you help your users to get there in different steps?
- How can you coach your users to this level through achieving different levels in games?

Practical example

Our nutritionist read the Scaling frame called jump across networks and realized that rather than promoting the concepts to schools herself, she could leverage existing networks that benefit from her concept. She made a long-list of these organizations, like health authorities, the ministry of education, the ministry of health and the farmers' association, and started reaching out to them to get them on board.

Call to action

Take 45 minutes with your team to go through each of the Scaling frames above and generate interventions to make your concept scale. Remember to postpone judgment and build on each other by saying yes and . . .

Tool 24: Waves Scaling Frames

For waves, we have identified four Scaling frames. These are all examples of how you can spot, create and harness energy around you to make your concept scale. These examples are not from the health care industry, but nonetheless, they can form inspiration for your project. Each Scaling frame consists of a description, an example and a set of trigger questions to guide your thinking.

Unleash a wave

Identify and unlock the existent pent-up energy within a system to create a movement or system that catalyzes your endeavor. Unlock this by removing a key constraint for society or by providing a focus and release to the energy, for instance through a major event or a movement (e.g. stage a rally or protest march). Make sure to tailor your communication to direct the momentum of the crowd. There is a tremendous amount of latent energy in most systems, since a portion of the population will always be dissatisfied with the way things are or has energy to spare.

Example:

- The Arab Spring is widely considered to have been sparked by the despair of Mohammed Bouazizi in Tunisia, which drove him to set himself on fire.
- Yet evidence shows that this event simply unlocked the pent-up frustration and anger experienced by populations across the MENA region, who endured increases in food prices and youth unemployment rates often reaching over 50%.

Trigger questions:

- Which widely shared frustration amongst your target user group is aligned with your cause? How could you reach these people credibly?
- What key constraint can you remove for society through your endeavor, thereby unleashing a wave of pent-up energy?

(continued)

(continued)

• Another example is the Canadian anti-consumerist, pro-environment magazine *Adbusters* initiating the call for a protest in Zurcotti Park in NY, which sparked the worldwide Occupy (Wall Street) movement – "we are the 99%."	• What event or messaging could you set up to focus the momentum of the unleashed crowd?

Catch a wave

Learn which underlying forces drive your window of opportunity, and be prepared to take full advantage of developments once such a wave appears. Like a surfer, look out for favorable external conditions, position yourself well and be prepared to catch the wave when the time is right. Put monitoring mechanisms in place to be able to react quickly.

Example:

- Collaborative consumption has become both a lifestyle and an industry segment within the last few years. Interest for the concept was sparked by a talk by Rachel Botsman at the TEDx Sydney conference in 2010, which she followed up with a bestselling book by Botsman and Rogers, *What's Mine Is Yours: The Rise of Collaborative Consumption*, and a prime time TV segment on the topic.

Trigger questions:

- What would ideally happen in the outside world – beyond your influence – that would drive your success?
- Where are your users already spending a lot of time and how would you redesign features or functions of your concept to benefit from this?

- The approach tapped into waves of a growing enthusiasm for sharing, coupled with a recession-driven need to reduce one's expenses on consumption. It has now turned into its own wave which got caught by hundreds of startups that support sharing of everything, from power drills to luxury cars, and from apartment renting to office space.

- How can you monitor potential new waves, what do you need to put into place to detect their weak signals?

Ride a wave

Nurture the wave you are riding and maintain your momentum by providing more energy, people and opportunities to those factors on which your success depends. Keep adapting your approach to changing conditions. Consider jumping on related waves to maintain relevance and reduce risks.

Example:

- Madonna has sold over 300 million records, making her the bestselling female recording artist of all time.
- She nurtured her wave of success by singing about topics defined by the zeitgeist, such as the NY underground dance style voguing, which in turn fueled the relevance of this zeitgeist- extending wave she had tapped into. She also cleverly associated herself with "hot" new artists (i.e. jumping on adjacent waves) and pushing creative boundaries.

Trigger questions:

- What are the pillar forces of the wave you are riding?
- How can you support these factors so they are maintained over a longer period of time?
- What adjacent waves can you jump on to maintain relevance and reduce risks?

Synchronize

Design synchronizing activities that give relevant
networks a heartbeat and a rhythm, with an
expectation of continuation over time, creating
a sense of synergy and common purpose.
Synchronization conditions the system to receiving
and carrying out messages or actions. A pulse gives
the system greater predictability, creating a sense of
confidence for participants that they have invested in
something that will be active in the long term. Once
a pattern has become established, it is likely to keep
being repeated.

Example:	Trigger questions:
• The *Star Wars* franchise was designed for synchronization, as the series of movies and their timing is carefully planned in advance, including the special approach of releasing a prequel trilogy as the second series.	• What could be recurring events, repeated activities on specific dates?
• The films of both trilogies were released at three-year intervals, with a range of related products like books, TV series, computer and video games and comic books marketed in the interim.	• What is the best time interval (rhythm) between events/activities? • How will regular communication be done, conditioning members of the network or system to receiving messages and carrying out actions?
• After the acquisition of creators Lucasfilm by Disney in 2012, fans were already being conditioned to await a new series of three movies, with the first one scheduled for release in 2015.	

Practical example

For the farmers' market in school idea, the team read the Scaling frame called catch a wave and realized that they could leverage the current trend of eating more healthy, local and organic. The team started coming up with ideas to hop on these trends, like allowing parents to buy from the farmers' market for their dinner and including more trendy words (like local, vegan, bio and organic) in their promotion materials.

Call to action

Take 45 minutes with your team to go through the Scaling frames above and generate interventions to make your concept scale. Remember to postpone judgment and build on each other by saying yes and . . .

Chapter 7

Creating Action

Now that you have been through the entire Innovation Flow, it's time to take your concept one step closer to reality; to create action. Creating Action is about generating momentum amongst the people around you so that they start helping to make your concept a reality. This chapter guides your entrepreneurial journey as you:

- identify the key stakeholders to involve in your concept going forward;
- develop an approach for each (group of) stakeholder(s);
- identify the elements of a pitch;
- develop your pitch. Create a workable pitch to infect others with enthusiasm about a product/idea;
- deliver your pitch.

At the end of this short chapter, you will understand the concept of pitching for action; you will have explored the required mind-sets and you will have worked on your challenge with tools from the Creating Action tool kit. You will conclude this chapter with a clearly identified set of stakeholders to involve and a concrete pitch.

Introduction to Creating Action

You have identified insights and user needs, and you have envisioned many ideas to settle on one concept that you prototyped and designed for scale. Now it's time to get more energy behind your concept. Creating Action is all about identifying who is key in making your concept a reality, developing strategies to involve them and creating a compelling story – or pitch – to involve them.

The goal of your stakeholder approach and pitch should be to generate enough interest to make someone want to set up a follow-up meeting or take a first step. External supporters or internal stakeholders within your places of work typically have significant responsibilities and many opportunities to spend their time. Your story must stand out by delivering a strong message that is interesting, engaging and tailored to their needs.

Having a solid pitch is as essential as having a good idea – you must "sell" your idea effectively. The goal of this chapter is to help you, the health entrepreneur, develop a clear, useful pitch that convinces your audience of the worth of your idea. In short, this chapter explores how to tell the story of your entrepreneurial concept in a compelling way. This chapter focuses on how to create and deliver a pitch that will motivate listeners to act and implement your idea. It's one thing to craft a pitch and an entirely different exercise to deliver the pitch in a way that is convincing and generates buy-in for your entrepreneurial idea. This chapter is a platform to practice both elements of your pitch.

With regards to top mind-sets, we've already discovered the required mind-sets in the previous chapters. When you're engaging stakeholders, you want to make them part of the story and feel some level of ownership. This means, you're effectively co-creating and prototyping with them. Therefore, the key mind-sets are:

- Yes and . . .: always encourage people to contribute to the concept by acknowledging their ideas (even the craziest) and by building on them. Celebrate failure: get feedback about what can still be improved and realize that people only provide feedback if they care.
- Iterate: there are always opportunities to improve, so allow your stakeholders to contribute and iterate the concept.

Review the Visioning and Prototyping chapters for more info on these mind-sets.

Challenge: start Creating Action

You've worked enough on your concept to bring it into the world for real! The rest of this chapter takes you through several practical tools to do so.

Tool 25: Stakeholder Engagement

To get something significant done in any ecosystem or organization, you need to understand who will support you, who will partner with you, who will resist you, how influential these players are and how motivated to do anything about it. To mobilize stakeholders at that scale, it is critical that you engage with all these people, at the right level, at the right time, in the right way, with the right message. Stakeholder Engagement therefore is a team effort, which requires explicit identification, mapping and action planning. The essence of Stakeholder Engagement is identify your stakeholders and consider how to meaningfully engage them.

Make a list of players that are affected by your concept and/or can affect the concept in any way; directly, indirectly, remotely. Map them on a two-by-two grid (low-high interest in outcome; low-high influence on outcome; green label for positive, red label for negative). For each, answer these questions:

- What (financial or emotional) interest do they have in the outcome of your concept, what is potential pain or gain?; how important is it to them? What motivates them most of all?
- What is the level of influence on successful outcome of your project; is their opinion positive or negative? Will they promote it or resist it?

For each of the four resulting domains, craft a meaningful approach that ranges from low intensity for the "Inform to Inspire" players and highest for the "Partner & Co-Create" players. Consider these questions:

- What support do you want from them?
- What information do they want from you?
- How do they want to receive information from you – what is the best way of communicating your message to them?

- If they are not likely to be positive what will win them round to give their support?
- If you are unlikely to win them around, then how will you manage their opposition?

Stay mindful that when you progress, the interest and influence field changes; continue to monitor and re-engage where needed.

Practical example

Our nutritionist mapped the key stakeholders around her.

She noticed that while the health of the children was key, they had little interest and influence over the concept coming to live or not. She also found out that while school boards should be interested in the project, they have so much on their plate that healthy eating doesn't always reach their list of priorities.

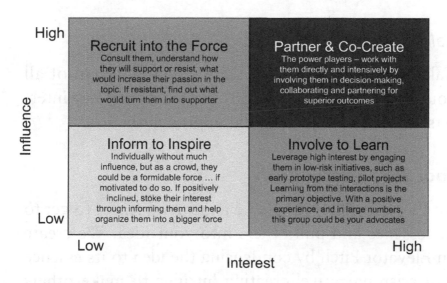

FIGURE 7.1 Stakeholder Engagement grid

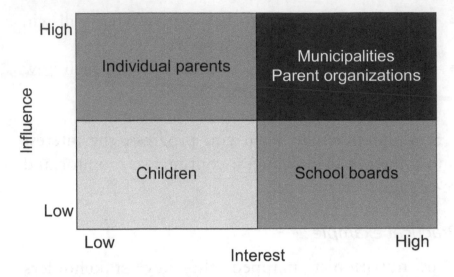

FIGURE 7.2 Stakeholder Engagement example

She proceeded to think about pitching to the municipality and parent organizations. What would be their key considerations to come on board, what could be their reasons not to do so and how could she partner and co-create with them?

Call to action

Take one hour with your team to build a map of all your stakeholders. Then consider what their key interests are and how you should approach them.

Tool 26: Elevator Pitch

An Elevator Pitch should be a gripping teaser to get to the essence and pull others into your idea. We create an Elevator Pitch by condensing the idea to its essence in a crisp narrative, creating intrigue to make others want to know more. You also want to craft a question for your audience that links to their position on the stakeholder grid and what you want them to do.

To create an Elevator Pitch, consider key ingredients like: vision, target user, user need, idea name, (market) category, key benefit, competitors and unique differentiator. Then craft the story to make it memorable. First, try this structure: [Idea Name] . . . is a . . . [Idea Categorization]. . . for . . . [Target User and User Need] . . . in a . . . [Delivery Method] that achieves . . . [Benefit] . . . E.g. *THNK is a school for mid-career professionals looking to enhance their creative leadership skills in a program with four intensive on-campus periods that readies them to lead their own innovation efforts.* When you have this essential structure, you can elaborate on it according to the circumstances, needs and target audience. Specifically, think back to the Stakeholder Engagement matrix and how you should edit your pitch for the four different quadrants.

When sharing it, always end with a question to pull people in to co-create with you. People will hear different things in your idea than you intended, but this can often make the idea richer. Questions you could ask would be: how would you describe this idea in your own words? What would you do to make this happen?

Practical example

After mapping her stakeholders, our nutritionist decided to pitch to the municipality for financial support and to the parent organizations for lobbying support toward the schools and local government.

She defined the essence of her pitch as: School Farmers' Market is a health intervention for parents and children in schools that makes eating more fruit and vegetables easy, educational and fun.

In pitching to the different stakeholders, she adapted her pitch. For example, to schoolboards she emphasized the fact that they didn't need to operate it themselves and asked them to be involved in prototypes. To municipalities, however, she emphasized the health benefits and asked them to co-create the solution with her.

Call to action

Take 45 minutes with your team to craft the essence of your pitch and adapt it for different stakeholders. You will continue to fine-tune your pitch based on the reactions of stakeholders; therefore, start with pitching to the less important stakeholders to allow yourself to learn.

Chapter 8

Conclusion

Go get 'em!

This book began with an explanation about why health professionals should be trained as entrepreneurs. We've provided real tools and resources for readers to build entrepreneurial solutions in the health care setting through approaches tested by nursing PhD candidates at George Washington University and by leaders from around the world at THNK School of Creative Leadership.

We trust that you will apply this approach coupled with your own ideas to innovate health care. Create an entrepreneurial solution to a pressing health care challenge. You know the challenges best, and now you have the tools necessary to design entrepreneurial solutions. Your solutions may not employ every part of the typical model for building a business. That's okay. Go ahead, tackle *that* problem that's been nagging at you for days, weeks, months or years. Do something about it. The opportunity to create positive change in health care is in your hands.

This book will have started to do its job when there is a clinical workforce empowered to address complex health care challenges and improve small things in their day-to-day work through entrepreneurship.

CONCLUSION: GO GET 'EM!

Entrepreneurship is an iterative process that involves continuous reflection and action. The real work entails acting on the enterprise business plan, reflecting on what worked or didn't and acting again. And again. And again with a bunch of pivots along the way.

There is not one right answer. It's every health care professional's job to uncover the most effective answer right now given the health information presented. Entrepreneurialism can be one useful avenue for achieving innovative approaches to excellent patient care. If you are ready to improve your patient's life, the organization you work in or perhaps even the world, there are several ways to go about it. One approach is health entrepreneurship.

References

Aron, E. N. (1996). *The highly sensitive person: how to thrive when the world overwhelms you*. New York: Carol Publishing.

Benammar, K. (2012, Nov. 11). *Reframing: the art of thinking differently*. Amsterdam: Uitgeverij Boom.

Catmull, E. (2008). *How Pixar fosters collective creativity*. Boston, MA: Harvard Business School Publishing.

Clark, R. W. (1971). *Einstein: the life and times*. New York: Avon Books.

Duverger, P. (2012). Variety is the spice of innovation: mediating factors in the service idea generation process. *Creativity and Innovation Management, 21*(1), 106–119.

Elkhorne, J. L. (1967, March). Edison: the fabulous drone – was Edison really a great genius? *73 Magazine, 78*, 52.

Eschleman, K. J., Madsen, J., Alarcon, G. & Barelka, A. (2014). Benefitting from creative activity: the positive relationships between creative activity, recovery experiences, and performance-related outcomes. *Journal of Occupational and Organizational Psychology, 87*(3), 579–598.

Frost, R. (1916). *Mountain interval*. New York: Henry Holt & Co. 17.

Giges, N. (2012, May). *Johannes Gutenberg*. Retrieved from www.asme.org.

Hilberts, B. (2018). *The Innovation Flow Toolkit, a manual for creating breakthrough vision and big ideas*. Retrieved from www.thnk.org/resources.

REFERENCES

Hilberts, B., van Dijk, M. & Benammar, K. (2014, Apr. 16). *Prototyping*. Retrieved from www.thnk.org.

Johnson, S. (2010). *Where good ideas come from: the natural history of innovation*. New York: Penguin Random House.

Mantel, H. (2010, Feb. 22). Hilary Mantel's rules for writers. *The Guardian*. Retrieved from www.theguardian.com.

Miró, J. & Lubar, R. (1964). *Joan Miró: I work like a gardener*. New York: Princeton Architectural Press.

Nooyen, L., Hilberts, B. & van Dijk, M. (2014, Apr. 16). *The process of visioning*. Retrieved from www.thnk.org.

Oppezzo, M. & Schwartz, D. L. (2014). Give your ideas some legs: the positive effect of walking on creative thinking. *Journal of Experimental Psychology: Learning, Memory and Cognition, 40*(4), 1142–1152.

Pavitt, N. (2016, March 25). *Brainhacking for beginners*. Retrieved from https://minutehack.com.

Pavitt, N. (2018, May 4). Generating the conditions for creativity to happen [Web log post]. Retrieved Oct. 29, 2018 from www.neilpavitt.com.

Powers, D. G. (1958). *How to say a few words effectively*. New York: Doubleday.

Prabahar, B. (2011, May 30). Is assumption the mother of all mistakes? [Web log post]. Retrieved Nov. 2, 2018 from https://blogs.sap.com.

Rich, C. (2016, Nov. 22). What are the key traits you look for when hiring an employee? *The Huffington Post*. Retrieved from www.huffingtonpost.com.

Ries, E. (2011). *The lean startup: how today's entrepreneurs use continuous innovation to create radically successful businesses*. New York: Crown Business.

Rosenberg, T. (2013, Jan. 16). A hospital network with a vision [Web log post]. Retrieved Nov. 2, 2018 from https://opinionator.blogs.nytimes.com.

Rozovsky, J. (2015, Nov. 17). The five keys to a successful Google team [Web log post]. Retrieved Nov. 2, 2018, from https://rework.withgoogle.com/blog.

Saint, N. (2009, Nov. 13). If you're not embarrassed by the first version of your product, you've launched too late. *Business Insider*. Retrieved from www.businessinsider.com.

Sawyer, K. (2017). *Group genius: the creative power of collaboration*. New York: Basic Books.

THNK School of Creative Leadership, www.thnk.org.org.

Turrell, M., van Dijk, M., Hilberts, B. (2014, Apr. 16). *Getting innovations to scale: networks*. Retrieved from www.thnk.org.

Umoh, R. (2018, Aug. 23). *The meeting hack loved by CEOs at Google, Facebook and LinkedIn*. Retrieved from www.cnbc.com.

van Asseldonk, T., van Dijk, M., Hilberts, B. & Turrell, M. (2014, Apr. 16). *Getting innovations to scale: emergence*. Retrieved from www.thnk.org.

van Dijk, M. & Hilberts, B. (2014, April 16). *Sensing is exploring uncharted territory*. Retrieved from www.thnk.org.

van Dijk, M., Hilberts, B. & Benammar, K. (2015, Nov. 4). *The serious job of prototyping*. Retrieved from www.innovationmanagement.se.

REFERENCES

Index

INDEX